Leishenshan Hospital
Guidelines for Nosocomial Infection Prevention and Control of COVID-19

雷神山医院新型冠状病毒感染院感防控指南

主 审　李六亿　林丽开
主 编　王行环　袁玉峰　茅一萍　乔 甫

U0349973

中国协和医科大学出版社

图书在版编目（CIP）数据

雷神山医院新型冠状病毒感染院感防控指南 / 王行环等主编 .— 北京：
中国协和医科大学出版社，2020.4
ISBN 978-7-5679-1244-1

Ⅰ.①雷… Ⅱ.①王… Ⅲ.①医院—感染—预防（卫生）—武汉—指南
②医院—感染—控制—武汉—指南 Ⅳ.① R197.323-62

中国版本图书馆 CIP 数据核字（2020）第 047075 号

雷神山医院新型冠状病毒感染院感防控指南

主　　编：王行环　袁玉峰　茅一萍　乔　甫
责 任 编 辑：许进力　高淑英
策 划 编 辑：崔　雨　张晶晶

出 版 发 行：**中国协和医科大学出版社**
　　　　　　（北京市东城区东单三条 9 号　邮编 100730　电话 010-65260431）
网　　　址：www.pumcp.com
经　　　销：新华书店总店北京发行所
印　　　刷：北京天恒嘉业印刷有限公司

开　　　本：710×1000　1/16
印　　　张：18.5
字　　　数：210 千字
版　　　次：2020 年 4 月第 1 版
印　　　次：2020 年 4 月第 1 次印刷
定　　　价：68.00 元

ISBN 978-7-5679-1244-1

雷神山医院新型冠状病毒感染院感防控指南
编写工作组

主　审　李六亿　林丽开

主　编　王行环　袁玉峰　茅一萍　乔　甫

副主编　朱小平　尚　东　刘志宇　张继东
　　　　王　莹

编　委　（按姓氏拼音排序）
　　　　冯毕龙　付　艳　傅小芳　甘　露
　　　　龚　斐　黄一乐　李　锟　李　敏
　　　　刘永宁　卢根娣　施　娣　王　鹏
　　　　王　婷　吴松杰　解　莹　翟桂兰
　　　　张红英　赵永娟　钟　倩　朱仕超

译　者　（按姓氏拼音排序）
　　　　陈　曦　陈怡然　高　翔　郭泳桦
　　　　蒋　翔　李恩成　李晶华　李晓勉
　　　　刘符生　刘颖懿　梅成杰　王岗岗
　　　　王坤雷　吴啸岭　许珂铨　闫凡芝
　　　　杨家钰　姚　烨　张　潇　张敏琪
　　　　祝逸民

Leishenshan Hospital Guidelines for Nosocomial Infection Prevention and Control of COVID-19

The Preparation of the Working Group

Translator(Sort by last name)

Xi Chen Yi–ran Chen Xiang Gao Yong–hua Guo
Xiang Jiang En–cheng Li Jing–Hua Li Xiao–mian Li
Fu–sheng Liu Ying–yi Liu Cheng–jie Mei Gang–gang Wang
Kun–lei Wang Xiao–ling Wu Ke–quan Xu Fan–zhi Yan
Jia–yu Yang Ye Yao Xiao Zhang Min–qi Zhang Yi–min Zhu

前　言

　　2020年新年伊始，新型冠状病毒肺炎便在神州大地上开始蔓延，来势汹涌，感染之快，牵动人心。从历史上看，抗击由病毒诱发的疫情，是人类发展过程中始终随行的一项艰巨任务。在未来，以新发突发重大传染性疾病为代表的非传统安全威胁是国际社会的共同敌人。疫情发生以来，党和政府高度重视，及时作出防控部署，全国动员、强力应对，采取了最全面、最严格的防控举措，打响了一场疫情防控的全民保卫战。在抗疫的关键时期，武汉雷神山医院，数天之内拔地而起，来自全国各地的十六支医疗队同舟共济、携手抗疫。虽然雷神山医院面临着边建设、边救治、边培训、边磨合的困难，但正是将所有工作人员健康安全放在至关重要的地位，才有了今日一个又一个的雷神山奇迹。应对不明原因的新发突发传染病，首要任务则是保护工作人员，因此本书的编写意在为全体医院工作人员提供来自雷神山医院感染防控的实战经验。

　　科学的环境布局与流程是有效防控的基础，因此，本书首先介绍具有雷神山医院特色与亮点的医院感染防控设计理念。在管理组织架构中，提出新建传染病医院感控工作开展的管理体系。在制度与流程中，依据国家防控方案的基本要求上，创造出了具有实际操作性的雷神山医院感控标准操作规程。在工作模式中，提出了三种雷神山医院感染防控日常高效工作模式。此外，还重点关注了院区内不同人群及驻地医疗队的医院感染防控问题。

　　目前，中国疫情防控形势持续向好，而世界多个国家和地区正处于疫情扩散期。在抗击疫情的过程中，医院感染管理责任重大，要确保医务人员在抗疫斗争中能够上得去、下得来、零感染，早日获得抗疫斗争的最终胜利。不驰于空想，不骛于虚声，有章可循，兢兢业业，脚踏实地，持之以恒，恪尽职守是雷神山医院每一位感控践行者的优秀品质的体现。本书编写时间有限，难免存在漏洞，敬请广大读者批评指正。最后，感谢所有奋战在抗疫战场的医务人员，正是他们的无私奉献使得我国赢得了与新型冠状病毒决战的阶段性胜利。

王行环　袁玉峰　茅一萍　乔　甫
2020 年 3 月 19 日于武汉雷神山医院

Preface

At the beginning of the New Year 2020, a novel coronavirus began to spread in the mainland of China, which had a strong impact on people's life. Historically, fighting epidemics of viruses has always been an arduous task in the continuum of human development. In future, non-traditional security threats such as outbreaks of major infectious diseases are expected to become public health enemies affecting the international community. Since the outbreak of the epidemic, the Party and the government have attached great importance to it, made timely prevention and control measures, implemented across the whole country. The Chinese government has adopted the most comprehensive and strict prevention and control measures, and initiated a national defense battle to ensure the spread of the epidemic of coronavirus is curtailed. During this epidemic period, Wuhan Leishenshan Hospital was rapidly constructed within a few days. More than 16 medical teams across the China joined hands to fight the epidemic. Despite the challenges encountered during the construction and operationalization of the Leishenshan Hospital, the most difficult task was ensuring the health and safety of all medical care personnel which has made the Leishenshan Hospital a miracle in the making. In response to new outbreaks of infectious diseases, the primary task is to protect the medical care personnel. Thus, the compilation of this book is intended to provide all hospital medical care personnel with actual combat experience needed to effectively prevent and control similar outbreaks based on experience from Leishenshan Hospital.

Scientific environmental layout and procedure are the basis for effective prevention and control. This book first introduces the conceptual design of nosocomial infection prevention and control based on the characteristics and highlights of Leishenshan Hospital. In terms of management and organization structure, the management system of the newly-built infectious disease hospital is proposed. For systems and procedures, a practical standard operating procedure of the Leishenshan Hospital has been created in line with the basic requirements of the national prevention and control plan. In the working mode aspect, three daily high-efficiency working modes employed in the Leishenshan hospital infection prevention and control are described. In addition, this book focuses on the prevention and control of nosocomial infection among different population cohorts and resident medical teams.

Currently, China's epidemic prevention and control situation is experiencing significant improvement, while many countries and regions in the world are in the period of rapid epidemic spread. In the process of fighting against the epidemic, the focus is on the management of nosocomial infections. It is important to ensure that medical personnel work and rest adequately and are not infected during the fight against the epidemic. Each medical personnel involved the Leishenshan Hospital high sense of focus, followed the rules, working conscientiously, high humility, perseverance, and completing their respective duties. Due to time constraints in the writing of this book, there are inevitable loopholes. Please feel free to criticize and correct the content of this book. Finally, we would like to thank all the medical personnel who were in the forefront of the battle against the epidemic. It was their selfless dedication that made our country achieve the staged victory in the decisive battle with the novel coronavirus.

Xing-huan Wang Yu-feng Yuan Yi-ping Mao Fu Qiao

专业名词释义

● **隔离**：采用各种方法、技术、防止病原体从患者及携带者传播给他人的措施。

● **负压隔离病房**：用于隔离通过和可能通过空气传播的传染病患者或疑似患者的病房。采用通风方式，使病房区域空气由清洁区向污染区定向流动，并使病房空气静压低于周边相邻相通区域空气静压，以防止病原微生物向外扩散。

● **清洁区**：病区中未受到患者血液、体液和病原微生物等物质污染及传染病患者不应进入的病区。

● **污染区**：病区中传染病患者和疑似患者直接接受隔离和诊疗的区域。

● **潜在污染区**：病区中位于清洁区与污染区之间，有可能被患者血液、体液和病原微生物等物质污染的区域。

● **缓冲间**：设置在清洁区与潜在污染区之间，潜在污染区与污染区之间的具有送机械通风措施的密闭室，双侧开门，其门具有互锁功能，不能同时处于开启状态。

● **终末消毒**：传染源离开疫源地后，对疫源地进行的一次彻底的消毒。如传染病患者出院、转院或死亡后，对病室进行的最后一次消毒。

● **手卫生**：洗手、卫生手消毒和外科手消毒的总称。

Definition

- Isolation: adoption of various methods and technologies to prevent the transmission of pathogens from patients and carriers to others.
- Negative pressure isolation ward: it is used to isolate patients with infectious diseases or suspected patients which pass through and may pass through the air. To prevent the spread of pathogenic microorganisms, the air in the ward area is forced to flow from the clean area to the polluted area, and the static pressure of the air in the ward is lower than that in adjacent areas.
- Clean area: the area that is not polluted with blood, body fluids, pathogenic microorganism and other substances from patients and should not be accessed by patients with infectious diseases.
- Polluted area: the area where infectious disease patients and suspected patients are directly isolated and treated.
- Potentially polluted area: this is the area located between the fish pollution areas in the clean area, which may be polluted with blood, body fluids, pathogenic microorganisms and other substances from patients.
- Buffer room: it is location between the clean area and the potentially polluted area, and between the potentially polluted area and the polluted area. It is a closed area that is fitted with mechanical ventilation measures. The doors are opened on both sides, and the doors are interlocked, and cannot be opened at the same time.
- Final disinfection: a thorough disinfection of the epidemic focus after the infectious source is removed from the area. For example, the final disinfection of the ward is done after discharge, transfer or death of the infectious disease patient.
- Hand hygiene: a general term for hand washing, hand disinfection and surgical hand disinfection.

目　录

Contents

图目录

Figure Datalogue

第一章　雷神山医院院区感染防控设计概述

第一节　雷神山医院的选址和感染防控设计原则

一、雷神山医院的选址

武汉雷神山医院是目前国内收治新型冠状病毒肺炎患者最多的传染病医院之一，也是国内最大的临时医院：医院占地面积328亩（21.9万平方米），房屋总建筑面积7.99万平方米，实际开放床位1423张，在院工作人员约3862人。雷神山医院位于武汉市江夏区黄家湖，北临军运路，东临黄家湖大道。医院建设参照战地医院形式，按照传染病医院标准设计，采用模块化、标准化安装和施工。

二、雷神山医院感染防控设计理念

（一）雷神山医院总体感染防控设计理念

从感染防控的设计理念来看，雷神山医院外围环境的设计要求为：隔离区与周边道路及建筑的间距至少20米的隔离带，满足传染病医院的要求。医院内感染防控设计主体思想为：医护、病患、物流交通流线明确、洁污分流、互不交叉（表1-1）。院区包括三大功能区域（图1-1）：医疗隔离区、医护生活区及保障功能区。

医疗隔离区分为南、北两区，北区包含 A 区 15 个病区、1 个 ICU、1 个手术室及 2 个医技区，南区包含 B 区 3 个病区、1 个 ICU 区和 C 区 12 个病区。所有病区均配备供氧系统、负压抽吸系统，可满足传染病医院各项功能。医疗隔离区内围设计理念为"鱼骨状"布局，"主骨"即为病区内医护主干道，从医护出入口进出，设有卫生通道；"分支"即为各隔离病房，每个隔离病房按照标准化病房单元打造，包括第一更衣室、第二更衣室、穿个人防护装备（personal protective equipment，PPE）房间、治疗室、护士站、配药室、医生办公室、洁净区内走道、缓冲区、隔离区内走道、标准化病室、外走道、仪器间、医疗废物暂存间、医生接待室、卫生处置间、标本存放间、茶水间等 18 个功能区域。

医护生活区包括医院办公楼、医护生活楼、清洁用品库及后勤区。医护生活区与医疗隔离区之间有 20 米的隔离绿化带。

保障功能区设有污水处理站、医疗废物焚烧站、医疗废物暂存点、正压站房、负压站房、液氧站、雨水收集池、救护车清洗消毒站等。

表 1-1　雷神山医院总平面设计考虑要素

分类	要求
环境	洁污、医患、人车等流线分区明确，动线清晰
建筑	建筑满足采光、卫生、通风、日照、消防等要求
环境保护	设有专门的医疗废物处理区域
感控	院区出入口 4 处
	患者主出入口处设救护车洗消场地

（二）雷神山医院负压隔离病房设计理念

为最大限度保证医患安全，雷神山医院隔离病房、医技科室及手术室均采用负压系统，病区内建筑结构密闭，在对气流进行精准控制下，不允许有自然通风的可能。负压隔离病房最小需要每小时 12 次换气，病室内与缓冲间的压差为 –10 ～ –5Pa，按病室厕所、病室、缓冲间、内走廊、缓冲间、办公区的顺序呈现梯度压力增加，使气流由清洁区流向潜在污染区再流向污染区，不允许倒流，每间病室，每个病室前缓冲间、内走廊均设有压力表，便于随时观察压力。

所有送风设置粗效、中效、亚高效空气过滤器三级过滤，送入洁净的空气，送风位置位于天花板。排风系统设置粗效、中效、高效空气过滤器三级过滤，阻隔病房内产生的灰尘和病原体，使排出空气符合生物安全和环境保护的要求，排风口设置在患者床头位置，排风口下边沿高于地面 0.1 米，上边沿不高于地面 0.6 米。

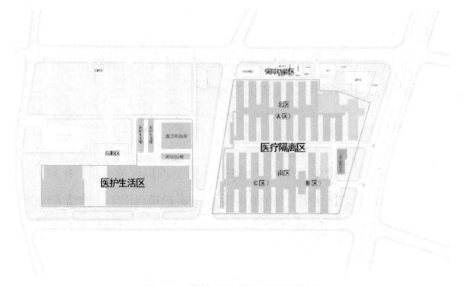

图 1-1　雷神山医院总平面设计图

第二节　雷神山医院院区布局流程

一、院区感染防控布局

整体看，雷神山医院院区的建筑布局完全符合传染病医院的"三区两通道"设计，严格分为清洁通道及污染通道，患者和医务人员出入口严格分开，清洁物品和污染物品出入口严格区分。清洁通道主要用于医护上下班通行，保洁、维修人员进出，清洁物资、清洗消毒后的被服和消毒后物品的传送等。污染通道主要用于患者通行、医疗废物转运、标本转运等。清洁通道与污染通道禁止逆行，从清洁通道进入污染通道时，必须穿戴 PPE，按照指定路线从事活动；在污染区工作的人员进入清洁通道时，必须经过 PPE 脱卸，手卫生通过后方可进入潜在污染区和清洁区（图 1-2）。

二、院区动线流程

清洁动线包括：全体工作人员（医务人员、内围保洁人员、维修人员等）上下班、清洁物资的进出等。所有的院区清洁区通道仅限于军体路 – 医务人员出入口 – 医护大街等。

污染动线包括：患者的进出、医疗废物转运、标本转运、救护车转运患者等。所有从病房出科的患者及其他污物，均从患者进出口出科，返回病区也一律从患者进出口返回。

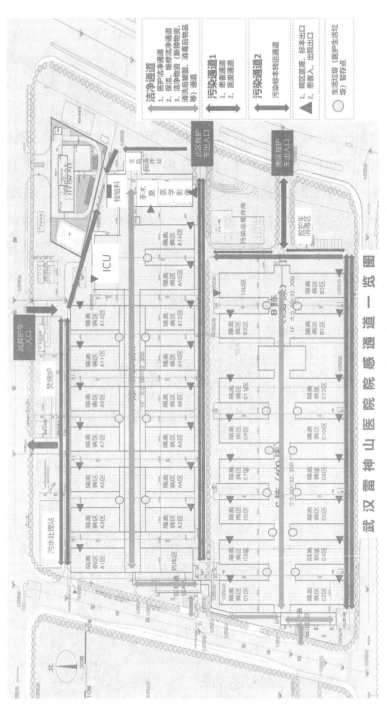

图1-2　雷神山医院院区通道图

第三节 雷神山医院病区感染防控布局流程

所有病区均为标准化单元建造，功能分区包括清洁区、潜在污染区及污染区。清洁区包括：医护休息室、值班室、沐浴更衣室、穿PPE房间。潜在污染区包括：护士站、物资通道、配药间、医生办公室及办公室外内走道、脱PPE房间等。污染区包括：隔离病室、患者外走道、污物暂存、污洗间等。各区之间设置缓冲间，不能同时双开门避免直接造成空气对流。在病室内、病室外缓冲间、医生办公室、护士站等区域均设置有洗手池，配置了自动感应的水龙头、洗手液、擦手纸、六步洗手法操作图、废纸篓等手卫生设施。病区布局图详见图1-3，病区主要动线流程见表1-2。

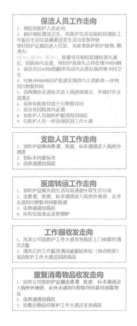
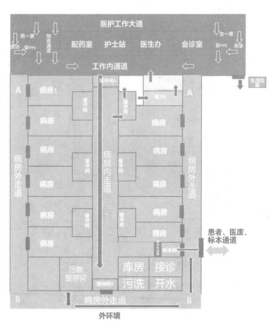

图1-3 雷神山医院病区布局图（箭头为流程动向）

表 1-2 雷神山医院院区动线流程（结合图 1-3）

人员	动线走向
医务人员	1. 医务人员上下班时，均由洁净通道即进入病区 2. 医务人员在外围活动时，穿戴 PPE，由患者通道进出
保洁人员	1. 上班时，按医护人员通道进入病区 2. 先做好清洁区和潜在污染区的清洁卫生 3. 穿好个人防护装备后，从脱防护装备的缓冲间逆向进入，先收集医护防护废物，顺序为缓冲 3→缓冲 2→缓冲 1，按要求在相应区域密封后，回病房内走道，将防护医疗废物先暂存在缓冲间 B 侧 4. 保洁员沿 A 向 B 的顺序完成内走道及病房缓冲间卫生 5. 经缓冲间 B 将防护医疗废物及病房内走道医疗废物一并转到污物暂存间 6. 由两侧外走道依次进入病房做清洁，并做好外走道清洁 7. 将所有医疗废物存放于污物暂存间 8. 保洁员回病房内走道 9. 按医护人员脱防护服流程回绿区 10. 同医护人员一样由绿区回工作大道
支助工作人员	1. 在清洁区穿防护装备进入病房外患者出入口处 2. 到患者出入口处标本间拿标本至检验科接收标本处 3. 由支助人员脱防护装备处脱卸防护装备回清洁区
医疗废物转运	1. 在医疗废物暂存间穿防护装备先到生活垃圾通道外取生活垃圾 2. 由患者、医疗废物、标本通道进入病房外通道，走外走道到污物暂存间取医疗废物 3. 由原通道出病区 4. 所有垃圾转运至焚烧炉
工作服收发	1. 洗涤公司人员由医护工作大道至各病区上门收取待清洗衣服 2. 清洗后的工作服由医护工作大道送回各病区
重复消毒物品	1. 消供公司穿防护装备由患者、医疗废物、标本通道进入病房外通道，走外走道到污物暂存间拿待消毒物品 2. 由原通道出病区 3. 消毒后物品经医护工作大道送至各病区

（乔甫　王莹　施娣　朱小平）

第二章　雷神山医院感染管理组织架构

第一节　组织架构

　　武汉雷神山医院建立了完整的医院感染管理组织架构体系，成立了医院感染管理委员会，由院长担任主任委员，主管医疗的副院长担任副主任委员，各医疗队领队为主要成员，并邀请国家卫生健康委员会派驻武汉的医院感染管理专家组成员担任顾问。医院感染管理委员会下设执行委员会，由主管医疗的副院长担任主任委员，院感组和各病区医院感染管理负责人担任委员（图2-1）。作为战时医院，武汉雷神山医院实行大部制管理，在医务管理部下设院感组、医务组、护理组、综合协调组等部门负责医疗服务工作。各病区医疗队，根据自身实际情况，均成立由科主任负责，护士长参与，感控专职人员组成的医院感染防控小组（图2-2）。

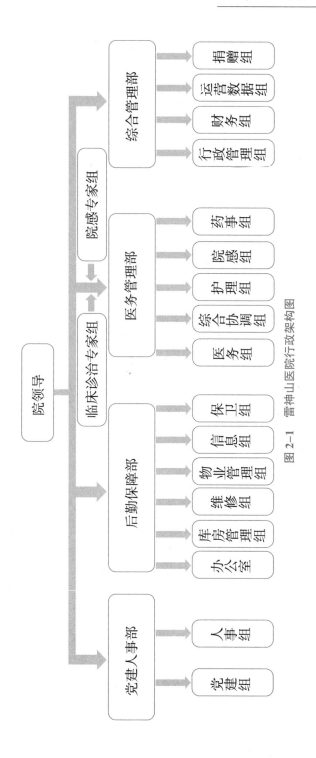

图 2-1 雷神山医院行政架构图

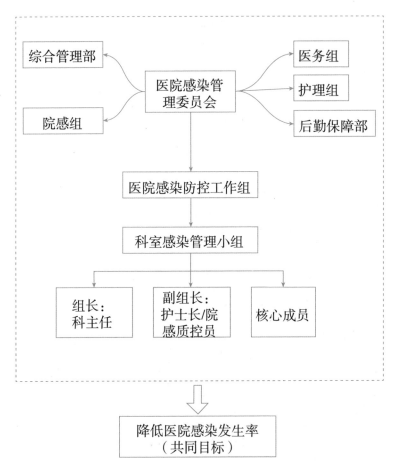

图 2-2 雷神山医院医院感染管理三级架构图

第二节 医院感染管理委员会职责

一、医院感染管理委员会依据国家的法律、法规，制定预防和控制医院感染防控的规划、标准、制度、监控措施及具体实施办法。

二、在新型冠状病毒肺炎防控期间，医院感染管理委员会对医院感染管理工作进行监督、检查、指导和咨询。

三、研究决定新型冠状病毒肺炎防控工作中医院感染应急工作的重大决策和重要事项，指挥调度医院各种资源力量参与医疗救治，决定启动、变更或终止医院应急响应级别。

四、医院感染管理委员会定期召开工作会议，总结工作、分析问题、布置任务，就存在问题及时向院领导及有关部门提出意见和建议，使医院感染防控预防与控制措施得到有效的落实。

五、负责协调全院各科室的医院感染防控工作，提供业务技术指导。

六、完成其他有关医院感染防控的重要事宜。

第三节 院感组人员组成及职责

一、人员组成

新建传染病医院医院感染防控管理办公室人员根据床位数合理配置。武汉雷神山医院计划 1500 张床位，按照每人管理 250 床配置 6 名院感防控人员。但由于雷神山医院建院初期面临着边建设、边接收患者的情况，因此院感组筹建初期从临床科室及其他部门紧急抽调人员，编制感染管理专职人员 13 名，在此基础上培养感染防控后备兼职人员 40 名。感染防控后备兼职人员经过为期 1 个月的理论与实践强化培训，主要承担各个病区感染防控督导员的职责。

二、工作职责

（一）在医院感染管理委员会的领导下，负责医院感染管理的日常工作。

（二）院感组按国家、省卫生健康委员会颁布的关于新型冠状病毒肺炎的医院感染防控和卫生学要求，对医院的建筑布局、重点科室的基本布局、基本设施和工作流程进行审查并提出指导意见。

（三）研究并确定医院感染防控重点部门、重点环节、重点流程、危险因素以及采取的干预措施，明确各有关部门、人员在医院感染防控工作中的责任。

（四）负责制定和颁布新型冠状病毒肺炎医院感染防控的有关规章制度，并监督检查其贯彻执行情况。

（五）负责新型冠状病毒肺炎医院感染防控宣传和所有医疗队医院感染培训。

（六）负责新型冠状病毒肺炎医院感染防控的规划并组织实施。

（七）定期向医院感染管理委员会汇报工作，研究、讨论、分析医院感染防控现状，以针对其感染因素（包括感染控制现状）部署工作、制定措施。遇有特殊情况，可随时紧急召集会议。

（八）定期对医院各科室环境、无菌物品管理、无菌技术操作环节、手卫生、消毒和隔离防护、重复使用医疗器械管理、医疗废物处置等进行监查，提出整改意见并督促整改落实。

（九）负责医务人员职业暴露的登记、指导、核查和防护。

第四节 临床科室医院感染管理小组构成及职责

一、按院感组的要求建立职责明确的临床科室医院感染管理小组，负责本科室的医院感染管理工作，明确小组人员职责并落实。

二、人员构成

（一）临床科室负责人为本病区医院感染管理第一责任人。

（二）科室医院感染管理小组成员包括医师和护士，设医院感染管理专职人员1名，为病区内相对固定人员。

三、职责

（一）临床科室医院感染管理小组负责本科室医院感染管理的各项工作，结合本科室医院感染防控工作特点，制定并组织实施相应的医院感染管理制度。

（二）配合医院感染管理部门进行本病区的新型冠状病毒肺炎和其他感染性疾病的监测和防控，定期对新型冠状病毒肺炎感染监测和防控工作的落实情况进行自查、分析，发现问题及时改进。

（三）负责对本科室固定、临时工作人员进行医院感染培训。

（四）接受医院对本科室医院感染管理工作的监督、检查与指导，落实医院感染管理相关改进措施，评价改进效果，做好相应记录。

四、医院感染质控员职责

（一）质控员由科室科主任、护士长在本科室内选定责任心和业务能力强、相对固定人员担任。建议科室安排其在科室内专职从事医院感染防控相关工作。

（二）在院感组、科主任、护士长的指导下，负责科室医院感染管理各项工作的落实。

（三）及时传达医院感染防控相关制度、流程和通知。参与制定并负责组织实施科室各项医院感染管理制度。

（四）对科室各项医院感染管理制度的执行情况进行督查与指导；指导配置各类消毒液，监控消毒液的浓度和质量。

（五）负责监督和指导医务人员、会诊人员、物流人员等的着装符合规范。

（六）负责科室各类医用防护装备、消杀药品及相关物品的及时领取与补充。

（七）进行医院感染防控知识、职业危害及防护措施知识培训；对新入科人员进行上岗前医院感染培训，培训均有记录。

（八）负责对卫生员进行清洁、消毒、隔离知识的培训并有记录，检查与指导卫生员清洁卫生工作的落实情况。

（九）及时向科主任、护士长反馈科室医院感染防控存在的问题。

（十）参加院感组组织的会议与培训，及时上交相关报表。

五、工作人员职责

（一）积极参加医院感染培训。

（二）遵守并落实医院感染管理委员会颁布的所有防护标准、规程及要求。

（三）开展新型冠状病毒肺炎医院感染的监测，按照医院的要求进行报告。

（四）了解新型冠状病毒肺炎医院感染防控相关知识。

（五）在从事无菌技术诊疗操作如注射、治疗、换药等时，应遵守无菌技术操作规程。

（六）遵循国家抗菌药物合理使用的管理原则，合理使用抗菌药物；监督并指导保洁员、安保员等掌握与本职工作相关的清洁、消毒与防护等知识和技能。

（朱小平　茅一萍　甘露　施娣）

第三章 医院感染防控制度
及标准操作规程

第一节 医院感染防控制度及应急预案

一、隔离病区医院感染防控制度

（一）应建立病区医院感染管理小组，负责病区医院感染管理工作，小组人员职责明确，并落实病区医院感染防控各项工作。

1. 管理要求　应建立职责明确的病区医院感染管理小组，负责病区医院感染管理工作，小组人员职责明确，并落实。

2. 人员构成

（1）病区负责人为本病区医院感染管理第一责任人。

（2）病区医院感染管理小组人员包括医师和护士。

（3）医院感染管理小组人员宜为病区内相对固定人员，医师宜具有主治医师以上职称。

3. 职责

（1）病区医院感染管理小组负责本病区医院感染防控及管理的各项工作，结合本病区医院感染防控工作特点，制定相应的医院感染防控管理制度，并组织实施。

（2）配合医院院感组进行本病区的医院感染防控监测，及时报告医院感染病例，并应定期对医感染监测、防控工作的落实情况进行自查、分析，发现问题及时改进，并做好相应记录。

（3）负责对本病区工作人员医院感染管理知识和技能的培训。

（4）接受医院对本病区医院感染管理工作的监督、检查与指导，落实医院感染管理相关改进措施，评价改进效果，做好相应记录。

4. 工作人员

（1）积极参加医院感染管理相关知识和技能的培训。

（2）遵守标准预防的原则，落实标准预防的具体措施，手卫生应遵循 WS/T 313 的要求；隔离工作应遵循 WS/T 311 的要求；消毒灭菌工作应遵循 WS/T 367 的要求。

（3）遵循医院及本病区医院感染防控相关制度。

（4）开展医院感染防控的监测，按照医院的要求进行报告。

（5）在从事无菌技术诊疗操作如注射、治疗、换药等时，应遵守无菌技术操作规程。

（6）保洁员、配膳员等应掌握与本职工作相关的清洁、消毒等知识和技能。

5. 教育与培训

（1）病区医院感染管理小组应定期组织本病区医务人员学习医院感染管理相关知识，做好考核。

（2）病区医院感染管理小组应定期考核保洁员的医院感染防控相关知识，如清洁与消毒、手卫生、个人防护等，根据其知识掌握情况开展相应的培训与指导。

（3）病区医院感染管理小组应对患者、陪护及其他相关人员进行医院感染防控相关知识如手卫生、隔离等的宣传及教育。

（二）工作要求

隔离病区的医院感染防控工作应按医院感染防控制度、病区消毒制度、病区医务人员防护制度、病区监测制度等开展工作。

1.病区布局合理，分区明确，保持环境整洁，定期清洁消毒。

2.非该病区工作人员原则上禁止入内，必须进入时，应经该病区医务人员许可，并接受隔离防护要求的指导，严格遵守隔离防护相关要求，做好登记记录。

3.医务人员进入病区内，应按工作区域要求做好相应防护，应保持衣帽整洁，操作时应严格执行无菌技术规程和手卫生相关制度。

4.医务人员应穿戴相应的个人防护装备（手套、口罩、帽子等），每诊治一位患者均应洗手或手消毒。个人防护装备每班次更换，遇污染时随时更换。

5.严格执行手卫生相关制度和要求，正确洗手，做好手卫生。

6.严禁穿戴工作区域的防护装备离开病区，外出应脱掉工作服或防护装备，穿戴个人衣物或外出服离开病区。

7.禁止探视患者。

二、医院感染监测制度

医院必须对患者开展医院感染监测，以掌握本院医院感染发病率、多发部位、多发科室、高危因素、病原体特点及耐药性等，为医院感染控制提供科学依据。

（一）医院应采取前瞻性监测方法进行全面综合性监测。

1.院感组必须每月对监测资料进行汇总、分析，定期向医院感染管理委员会、医院感染管理工作委员会书面汇报，向全院医务人员反馈，监测资料应妥善保存，特殊情况及时汇报和反馈。

2.对医院感染进行暴发预警监测，及时发现问题，向分管院长进行汇报。

3. 医院应监测除新型冠状病毒肺炎以外的疾病，如有传染性疾病应按传染病管理要求及时上报。

4. 逐步通过医院感染信息化开展监测，定期对监测资料进行趋势分析。

（二）医院应在全面综合性监测的基础上开展目标性监测，监测目标根据本院的特点、医院感染防控的重点和难点决定。

（三）应定期对目标监测资料进行分析、反馈，对其效果进行评价及提出改进措施；应有阶段性总结报告；监测结束，应有终结报告。

（四）医院必须对消毒效果定期进行监测。灭菌合格率必须达到100%，不合格物品不得进入临床使用部门。

（五）环境卫生学监测：包括对空气、物体表面和医护人员手的监测。

（六）各病区应严格按《武汉雷神山医院医院感染防控监测指南》的要求开展各项监测，详见附录1。

三、隔离病区医院感染监控专职人员工作制度

（一）在院感组及科室护士长指导下，监督本科室医院感染防控制度、消毒隔离制度、无菌操作常规等的落实，日工作要细化到具体项目及项目可能完成的时间，并记录。

（二）对疑似或确诊医院感染病例，监督医师及时通过内网"感染管理软件"信息系统上报，并尽可能留取相应标本送细菌学检查及药敏试验。如发现在诊疗过程中短时间内出现3例以上临床症状相同或相近的感染病例，尤其是病例间可能存在具有流行病学意义的共同暴露因素或者共同感染来源时，无论有无病原体同种同源检测的结果或检测回报结果如何，都应及时向本科室医院感染管理小组负责人报告，医院感染管理小组负责人立即电话报告院感组和医务组，协助做好流行病学调查，调查发病原因，积极采取控制措施。

（三）监督检查病房日常消毒、终末消毒、传染与感染患者的隔离消毒管

理情况；做好高危易感人群的保护性隔离。

（四）负责督查无菌技术操作及消毒隔离工作质量及手卫生执行情况，监督检查病房配置和使用消毒药械情况及一次性医疗用品使用和处理情况。

（五）按院感组计划安排做好本科室的空气、物体表面、医务人员手等的监测工作，并做好记录。

（六）至少每周1次完成紫外线灯管的清洁。

（七）对使用中消毒液浓度进行监测并记录，对浓度不达标的消毒液应及时更换（含氯消毒液应每日监测）。

（八）指导并督查病区保洁员的日常清洁消毒及医疗废物交接登记等工作。

（九）围绕本科室医院感染管理的质量指标进行月质控。

（十）负责落实本科室的医院感染防控知识宣传，并组织科内人员参加有关医院感染培训。

（十一）至少每月1次对各项医院感染监测、监管结果进行总结、分析和反馈并持续改进，归档、备查。

四、隔离病区日常清洁消毒制度

（一）病区内常规清洁消毒规范

1.医务人员工作时间应衣帽整洁，严格遵守无菌技术操作规程，严格执行手卫生规范，不得穿工作服进入餐厅、宿舍和医院外环境。

2.正确使用消毒剂、消毒器械、一次性无菌医疗用品等。一次性无菌医疗用品用后按医疗废物处置。

3.凡接触皮肤、黏膜的器械和用品必须达到消毒要求；凡进入人体组织或无菌器官的医疗用品必须达到灭菌要求。

4.抽出的药液放置不得超过2小时，开启的无菌溶液必须在2小时内使用，各种溶媒启封后不得超过 24 小时，并注明开启时间。

5. 开启使用的碘酒、酒精随用随关，每周更换。纸塑包装的灭菌物品（棉签、棉球、纱布）一经打开，保存时间不超过 4 小时。锐器盒开启时间不能超过 48 小时。

6. 使用的清洁工具（抹布、地巾等）标识明确，分别清洗，定点放置，定期消毒，不得交叉使用。

7. 病床湿扫（一床一巾）、床头柜湿抹（一柜一巾），使用后浸泡消毒。患者出院、转科、死亡后应对患者的床单位进行终末消毒。

（二）具体实施方法

1. 病区日常清洁消毒由本病区护理人员及保洁人员共同负责，护理组每日应设有消毒班，专门负责指导当班保洁人员个人防护，并协助保洁人员共同完成当日清洁消毒工作，病区护士长负责督导落实。

2. 应尽量选择一次性诊疗用品，非一次性诊疗用品应首选压力蒸汽灭菌，不耐热物品可选择化学消毒剂或低温灭菌设备进行消毒或灭菌。

3. 配置含氯消毒液

（1）含氯消毒剂泡腾片（每片 500mg）配制成有效氯 1000mg/L 的含氯消毒液。

（2）配置方法：1L 水加入 2 片（每片 500mg），6L 水加入 12 片（每片 500mg）。

（3）消毒液配制好后应使用消毒剂浓度试纸进行有效浓度的监测并记录，监测合格方能使用。注意事项：含氯消毒剂应现配现用，使用时间不能超过 24 小时。

4. 物体表面、地面应定时清洁及消毒，每日 2 次；遇污染时随时进行消毒处理。

5.消毒方法

（1）室内空气的消毒在无人条件下打开紫外线灯进行，用紫外线消毒时，可适当延长照射时间到1小时以上。

（2）应遵循先清洁再消毒的原则，采取湿式卫生的清洁方式。

（3）清洁病房或诊疗区域时，应有序进行，由上而下，由里到外，由轻度污染到重度污染；有多名患者共同居住的病房，应遵循清洁单元化操作。

（4）物体表面用能达到高水平消毒的湿巾进行擦拭消毒，地面采用1000mg/L的含氯消毒液或500mg/L的过氧化氢消毒剂消毒，消毒作用时间应不少于30分钟。

（5）在诊疗过程中发生患者体液、血液等污染时，应随时进行污点清洁与消毒。

（6）病区的标本存放箱应用1000mg/L的含氯消毒剂擦拭内、外表面，每日1次。

（7）医疗废物应遵循《医疗废物管理条例》和《医疗卫生机构医疗废物管理办法》的要求，规范使用双层黄色垃圾袋封装放至医疗废物暂存间，医疗废物集中处置的工作人员再套一层黄色垃圾袋将医疗废物运送至医疗废物焚烧站集中处理。

（8）使用后的清洁工具处理：抹布及拖把，应分别在1000mg/L的含氯消毒剂中浸泡消毒30分钟，清洗干净，晾干备用。清洁车，用后推回处置间，用1000mg/L的含氯消毒剂擦拭车身后清水擦拭，去除残留的消毒剂备用。

五、隔离病区终末消毒制度

（一）消毒时机

终末消毒是指传染源离开有关场所后进行的一次彻底的消毒，如患者出院、转科、死亡后进行的病房空气、物体表面及地面的消毒。应确保终末消毒后的场所及其中的各种物品不再有病原体的存在。终末消毒对象包括患者排出的污染物（血液、分泌物、呕吐物、排泄物等）及其可能污染的一切用具（包括医疗、护理用品）和环境，不必对室外环境（包括空气）开展大面积消毒。

（二）消毒流程

常规擦拭清洁消毒，根据情况行紫外线消毒。

（三）执行人员

工作区域的在岗医务人员负责本区域的终末消毒工作，具体执行人员科室指派。

（四）消毒方法

1.空气　无人条件下可选择 0.2% 过氧乙酸、500mg/L 二氧化氯、3% 过氧化氢消毒剂，按照 10～20ml/m³ 的用量，进行超低容量喷雾消毒，作用 1 小时。

2.地面、墙壁　有肉眼可见污染物时，应先完全清除污染物再消毒。无肉眼可见污物时，可用 1000mg/L 的含氯消毒液擦拭或喷洒消毒。消毒作用时间应不少于 30 分钟。

3.物体表面

（1）一般物体表面有肉眼可见物时，应先去污再消毒。

（2）个人电子产品可选用 75% 酒精或含双链季铵盐的卫生纸巾擦拭消毒。

（3）床架、床头柜、家具、呼叫器、玩具、病床摇柄、门把手、水龙头、洗手池、马桶按钮、坐垫及内外表面等用含有效氯 1000mg/L 的含氯消毒液或 500mg/L 的二氧化氯消毒液等擦拭、喷洒消毒。多组件组合的物品，如床头柜，应打开抽屉和柜门，对内外表面都应喷洒或擦拭到位，作用30分钟后清水擦拭干净。

（4）呼吸机、ECMO、CT机、监护仪等贵重设备，应按照各自相应规程或说明书进行处理、其他诊疗设备，如体温计、听诊器、输液泵、血压计、血氧仪、除颤仪等设备表面，可根据具体物品是否耐腐蚀，灵活选用75%酒精、1000mg/L的含氯消毒液或500mg/L的二氧化氯等擦拭、浸泡、喷洒消毒。作用30分钟后清水擦拭干净。

4. 污染物（患者血液、分泌物、呕吐物和排泄物） 少量污染物可用一次性吸水材料（如纱布、抹布等）沾取5000～10 000mg/L的含氯消毒液（或能达到高水平消毒的消毒湿巾或干巾）小心移除。大量污染物应使用含吸水成分的消毒粉或漂白粉完全覆盖，或用一次性吸水材料完全覆盖后用足量的5000～10 000mg/L的含氯消毒液浇在吸水材料上，作用30分钟以上（或能达到高水平消毒的消毒干巾）小心清除干净。清除过程中避免接触污染物，清理的污染物按医疗废物集中处置。

5. 织物的处理 患者使用后的床单、被罩等织物进行双层医疗废物袋密闭封装，按照感染性医疗废物焚烧。有条件的病区可使用床单位消毒机进行消毒。

6. 医疗用品 尽量使用一次性诊疗器械、器具和物品，使用后应进行预处理，随后用双层医疗废物袋密闭封装，按照感染性医疗废物处置，可复用诊疗器械用双层医疗废物袋盛装，贴上标签，放整理箱内联系消毒供应中心处理。

7. 医疗废物 应遵循《医疗废物管理条例》和《医疗卫生机构医疗废物管理办法》的要求，规范使用双层黄色医疗废物收集。盛装的医疗废物达到包装的3/4时，进行紧实严密地封口，在隔离区的污染物暂存间喷洒消毒或再套一层黄色医疗废物袋将医疗废物运送至焚烧站。

8. 患者个人物品 患者不需要带走的物品建议均按照医疗废物集中焚烧

处理。其他需要带走的个人物品无肉眼可见污染物时，若需重复使用，可先用 500mg/L 的含氯消毒液浸泡 30 分钟，然后按常规清洗。其他随身用品可用紫外线照射 1 小时或者耐湿的物品可用 1000mg/L 含量消毒剂浸泡消毒 30 分钟。患者的衣物，可用紫外线里外各照射 1 小时以上，之后密封保存 14 周后再用。

9. 尸体处理　患者死亡后，要尽量减少尸体移动和搬运，应由经培训的工作人员在严密防护下及时进行处理。用 3000 ~ 5000mg/L 的含氯消毒剂棉球或纱布填塞患者口、鼻、耳、肛门、气管切开处等所有开放通道或创口；用浸有消毒液的双层布单包裹尸体，装入双层尸体袋中，由民政部门派专用车辆直接送至指定地点尽快火化。

六、新型冠状病毒肺炎医疗废物管理制度

（一）医疗废物主要是从各隔离病区、治疗室、检验科等新型冠状病毒肺炎患者生活垃圾及污染区所产生的一切废物。

（二）分为感染性医疗废物、病理性医疗废物、化学性医疗废物、药物性医疗废物、损伤性医疗废物。

（三）用黄色垃圾袋封装（3/4）；锐器使用利器盒封装（3/4）。

（四）黄色垃圾袋进行密封打包双层包装：鹅颈式分层包扎用扎线带封口贴标签：包括产生医院及科室、产生日期、类别（标注是新型冠状病毒肺炎）、重量，袋数。

（五）交接签字。病区与转运人员进行称重，外套第三层黄色医疗废物袋或喷洒消毒液（1000mg/L）交接并双签字留存。

（六）进行运送（按指定路线转运），且不能和生活垃圾混合运送至医疗废物暂存处暂存并做好交接记录。

（七）由医院焚烧炉统一进行焚烧。

七、职业暴露管理制度

（一）医务人员预防新型冠状病毒肺炎感染和其他各类感染性疾病的防护措施应当遵照标准预防原则，对所有患者的血液、体液及被血液、体液污染的物品均视为具有传染性的病原物质，医务人员接触患者和这些物质时，应采取防护措施。

1. 接触新型冠状病毒肺炎患者或进入隔离病区工作时，应按相关要求流程做好个人防护，包括穿戴医用防护口罩、一次性帽子、医用防护服、乳胶手套、靴套、防护面屏或护目镜等防护装备。

2. 在诊疗、护理操作过程中，有可能发生血液、体液大面积喷溅或者有可能污染医务人员的身体时，应加穿具有防渗透性能的隔离衣或者防水围裙。

3. 医务人员手部皮肤发生破损，在进行有可能接触患者的血液、体液的诊疗和护理操作时应戴双层手套。

4. 医务人员在进行侵袭性诊疗、护理操作过程中，要注意防止针头、缝合针、刀片等锐器刺伤或者划伤。

5. 使用后的锐器应当直接放入耐刺、防渗漏的锐器盒，禁止回套针帽，禁止用手直接接触使用后的针头、刀片等锐器。

（二）医务人员发生职业暴露后，应先评估暴露风险，然后按相应流程处置：

1. 高暴露风险　面对确诊患者直接暴露时，包含以下情况：

（1）皮肤暴露：被大量肉眼可见的患者体液、血液、分泌物或排泄物等污物直接污染皮肤。

（2）黏膜暴露：被肉眼可见的患者体液、血液、分泌物或排泄物等污物直接污染黏膜（如眼睛、呼吸道）。

（3）针刺伤：被直接接触了确诊患者体液、血液、分泌物或排泄物等污物的锐器刺伤。

（4）呼吸道直接暴露：在未戴口罩的确诊患者1米范围内口罩脱落，露出口或鼻。

2.低风险暴露　未直接暴露，即防护装备破损或脱落或接触皮肤，包含以下情况：

（1）手套破损：手套破损，未发生肉眼可见的污物直接接触皮肤。

（2）外层防护装备接触皮肤或头发：主要是脱防护装备时，外层污染的防护装备接触了皮肤或头发。

（3）防护服破损：防护服破损，未发生肉眼可见的污物直接接触皮肤。

（4）呼吸道间接暴露：在患者1米以外或佩戴口罩的患者面前口罩脱落。

3.处置　详见隔离区高风险暴露时处置流程和隔离区低风险暴露时处置流程。

（三）后期干预

1.一旦发生职业暴露，进行应急处理后，立即上报科主任或护士长，并上报雷神山医院院感组。

2.可酌情在医师指导下服用抗病毒药进行预防，应给予随访和咨询，并进行必要的针对性暴露者新型冠状病毒的核酸变化监测，对服用药物的毒性进行监控和处理，观察和记录相关感染的早期症状等。

3.院感组负责对职业暴露情况进行登记。登记内容包括：职业暴露发生时间、地点及经过；暴露方式；暴露的具体部位及损伤程度、暴露源种类情况；处理方法及处理经过，是否实施预防性用药及用药依从性情况；定期检测及随访情况。

4.各病区和医院院感组，定期将职业暴露情况进行汇总分析，并根据分析结果采取有效整改措施，持续做好医务人员职业防护。

八、手卫生管理制度

（一）全体医务工作者应严格按照本制度要求做好手卫生。科主任及护士长要带头执行医务人员的手卫生规范。各科室每月开展本科室手卫生依从性相关自查，力争做到手卫生依从性及正确率的持续改进。

（二）全院必须配备合格的手卫生设备和设施，手消毒剂的包装和洗手后的干手物品（毛巾）或设施应避免造成二次污染。

（三）所有医务人员必须掌握正确的手卫生方法，保证洗手与手消毒效果。

（四）医务人员正确掌握洗手及手消毒指征。

（五）医务人员手无可见污染物时，可用快速手消毒剂消毒双手代替洗手。

（六）医务人员手被可见污染物污染以及直接为传染病患者进行检查、治疗、护理或处理传染病患者污染物之后，应先用流动水冲净，然后使用手消毒剂消毒双手。

（七）手卫生指征

1.直接接触患者前后，接触不同患者之间，从同一患者身体的污染部位移动到清洁部位时。

2.接触患者黏膜、破损皮肤或伤口前后，接触患者的血液、体液、分泌物、排泄物、伤口敷料之后。

3.穿脱防护装备前、中、后。

4.进行无菌技术操作前后，处理清洁、无菌物品之前，处理污染物品之后。

5.当医务人员的手有可见的污染物或者被患者的血液、体液污染后。

6.接触患者周围环境后。

九、应急预案管理制度

（一）每天对医院工作人员体温进行监测和上报，及时登记呼吸道、消化道等可疑感染症状等情况的工作人员，并持续追踪。

（二）对体温异常并有可疑症状的工作人员，及时隔离并立即上报院感组及保健科，由保健科完善相关检查，同时排查密切接触者。

（三）严格执行《职业暴露处理流程》，在工作中一旦发生职业暴露，按照相关流程进行处理。

（四）严禁任何工作人员在发生职业暴露和发热伴呼吸道症状感染时瞒报、谎报，在隔离期间服从医院统一管理和安排。

十、可复用诊疗器械 / 物品管理制度

（一）医院所有病区可重复使用的诊疗器械 / 物品应按相关操作流程规范处理，统一由物业公司进行回收、清洁、消毒 / 灭菌处理后再次使用，任何科室和个人不得私自处理。

（二）新型冠状病毒肺炎患者使用后的可复用诊疗器械 / 物品应遵循消毒 – 清洁 – 消毒 / 灭菌的原则。

（三）各病区使用后的可复用诊疗器械 / 物品，应首先在病区污洗间进行消毒预处理，封装在双层黄色垃圾袋中湿式存放，粘贴标识，交接后交由物业回收人员。

（四）消毒预处理建议使用含氯消毒剂，有效氯含量 1000mg/L。

十一、感染性织物管理制度

收集时应动作缓慢，避免产生气溶胶。若未一次性使用的，按照医疗废物集中焚烧处理。若需重复使用，床单、被套、枕套等织物可采用流通蒸汽或煮

沸消毒 30 分钟，或用含氯消毒液 500mg/L 浸泡 30 分钟。棉絮、被芯、枕芯、床垫等可采用 1000mg/L 含氯消毒液或 500mg/L 二氧化氯消毒液喷洒至表面湿润，作用 1 小时后晾干。有条件的病区，可采用床单位消毒机进行消毒。

十二、全体人员健康管理制度

（一）维护医院工作人员职业安全，有效预防医院工作人员在各项工作中出现职业危害，保护工作人员身体健康。

（二）医院工作人员包括医疗、护理、医技、药学、行政、后勤等所有部门人员，在工作期间均享受医院医疗安全保障。

（三）医院对职业危害的预防以落实职业病防治法实行预防为主的原则，为所有工作人员提供整洁的工作环境、合理的工作流程和必要的防护装备等。

（四）加强工作人员在工作时的安全教育。上岗前必须进行感染防控相关知识和技能，尤其是职业防护的培训。

（五）各病区应对所有工作人员进行每日健康监测，包括体温和其他呼吸道感染症状监测、消化道监测、皮肤破损监测等，做好登记和随访工作。

（六）应按相关流程对工作人员进行定期体检，如发生感染或疑似感染应尽快上报并隔离治疗，同时做密切接触者的追踪随访调查。

十三、治疗室感染管理制度

（一）非工作人员不得入内，医务人员进入室内应衣帽整洁，操作时应严格执行无菌技术规程和手卫生要求。

（二）无菌物品与非无菌物品、清洁物品与污染物品应分开放置，标识清楚；治疗车的上层为清洁区，下层为污染区。

（三）保持室内整洁，每日 2 次湿式清洁及消毒物体表面及地面，物体表面用高水平的消毒湿巾擦拭，地面用 1000mg/L 含氯消毒液拖擦，作用 30 分钟；如遇污染应随时清洁消毒；每日 2 次使用空气消毒机进行空气消毒，每次 1 小时，并记录。

（四）开启的无菌溶液应在 2 小时内使用；各种溶媒、外用生理盐水、高渗盐水无菌棉签一经启用，使用时限不得超过 24 小时。

（五）严格按照医疗废物管理的相关制度、规定落实医疗废物的管理。

（六）每班次上班后由治疗室负责护士进行治疗室环境和空气消毒。

十四、防护装备使用指引

为进一步做好雷神山医院的新型冠状病毒肺炎预防与控制工作，有效杜绝新型冠状病毒的传播风险，规范医务人员行为，结合新型冠状病毒的病原学特点、传染源、传播途径、易感人群等以及传染病医院工作特点，特制定本指引，方便大家执行。医疗机构应当根据医务人员在工作时接触新型冠状病毒肺炎疑似患者或确诊患者的可能性，按照导致感染的危险程度采取分级防护，防护措施应当适宜（附录 5）。主要有以下几种防护级别。

（一）一般防护

1. 严格遵守标准预防的原则。

2. 工作时应穿工作服、戴医用外科口罩。

3. 认真执行手卫生。

（二）一级防护

1. 严格遵守标准预防的原则。

2. 严格遵守消毒、隔离的各项规章制度。

3. 工作时应穿工作服、隔离衣，戴工作帽和医用外科口罩，必要时戴乳胶手套。

4. 严格执行手卫生。

5.离开隔离区域时进行个人卫生处置，并注意呼吸道与黏膜的防护。

（三）二级防护

1.严格遵守标准预防的原则。

2.根据传播途径，采取飞沫隔离与接触隔离。

3.严格遵守消毒、隔离的各项规章制度。

4.进入隔离病房、隔离病区的医务人员必须戴医用防护口罩，穿工作服、隔离衣和／或医用防护服、鞋套，戴手套、工作帽，必要时戴护目镜或防护面屏。严格按照清洁区、潜在污染区和污染区的划分，正确穿戴和脱摘防护装备，并注意口腔、鼻腔黏膜和眼结膜的卫生与保护。

（四）三级防护

三级防护是在二级防护基础上，加戴正压头套或全面型呼吸防护器。

十五、武汉雷神山医院医院感染暴发控制应急预案

（一）目的

为预防、控制和消除发生在我院的医院感染暴发及其造成的危害，指导和规范医院感染暴发的应急处置工作，保护患者和医务人员身体健康，根据《中华人民共和国传染病防治法》《突发公共卫生事件应急条例》《医院感染管理办法》《医院感染暴发报告及处置管理规范》《医院感染监测规范》等法律法规的规定，结合本院实际，制定本预案。

（二）适用范围

本预案适用于武汉雷神山医院医院感染暴发或疑似暴发的应急处理工作。

（三）医院感染暴发的定义、分级

1. 定义

（1）医院感染暴发：指在医疗机构或其科室的患者中，短时间内发生 3 例以上同种同源感染病例的现象。

（2）疑似医院感染暴发：指在医疗机构或其科室的患者中，短时间内出现 3 例以上临床综合征相似、怀疑有共同感染源的感染病例；或者 3 例以上怀疑有共同感染源或感染途径的感染病例现象。

2. 分级

Ⅰ级：①10 例以上的医院感染暴发事件；②发生特殊病原体或者新发病原体的医院感染；③可能造成重大公共影响或者严重后果的医院感染。

Ⅱ级：①5 例以上医院感染暴发；②由于医院感染暴发直接导致死亡；③由于医院感染暴发导致 3 人以上人身损害后果。

Ⅲ级：发生 3 例以上医院感染暴发或 5 例以上疑似医院感染暴发。

（四）应急组织机构与职责

医院成立医院感染暴发应急领导小组，领导小组下设应急办公室，其职责和人员分别如下：

1. 医院感染暴发事件领导小组

（1）职责：研究并制定发生医院感染暴发事件时的控制方案；发生医院感染流行或暴发趋势时，负责对本院的医院感染暴发成立与否做出最终判断；负责统筹协调组织相关科室、部门开展医院感染暴发的调查与控制工作，并按要求报告有关卫生行政部门。

（2）人员组成：

组长：一人

副组长：若干

成员：若干（包括各医疗队总负责人）

2.医院感染暴发处置应急办公室（挂靠医务管理部院感组）

（1）职责：具体负责落实领导小组的各项工作决议，督促我院按应急预案开展工作，落实各项处置措施组织实施、协调督办信息报告、通报、疫情上报等工作，在突发公共卫生事件应急防治工作中，全院各临床医技科室、行政及后勤保障部门必须服从防治工作办公室的统一协调和调度指挥。

（2）人员组成：

办公室主任：一人

办公室成员：若干（包括各医疗队感染防控负责人）

秘书：一人

（五）医院感染暴发的监测与报告

1.各病区应按医院的总体要求，对医院感染暴发开展主动监测，应急办加强监测工作的管理和督导，保证监测质量，具体如下：

（1）全院建立院感组、检验科、各病区医院感染管理小组三位一体的监控反馈网络，提高疑似医院感染暴发的发现和监控处理的应急能力。

（2）完善的医院感染病例会诊制度：当发现医院感染暴发趋势而需要对感染病例进行会诊或核实诊断时，由医务组负责组织相关专家完成病例会诊或核实诊断的工作。

2.各病区遇有以下报告内容情形之一，立即向院感组报告（下班时间报院总值班）。

（1）主管医生和感控护士发现科室短时间内出现3例以上同种病原体感染，由主管医生初步判断是否为医院感染暴发，若"是"或"高度疑似"立即报告科室主任，主任组织人员对上述病例进行核查，再次判断是否为医院感染暴发，若仍然判断为"是"或"高度疑似"则及时电话报告院感组。

（2）院感组医院感染散发病例监测人员以及片区管理人员发现同一科室短时间内出现3例以上具有相同综合征的医院感染，立即到达现场进行流行病学调查，根据感染暴发事件情况，汇报医院感染管理委员会，并按要求进行报告。

（3）报告内容按照国家、省级卫生行政部门规定分为首次报告、进程报告和结案报告，根据事件的严重程度、事态发展和控制情况及时报告事件进程。

（4）任何科室或个人对医院感染暴发事件不得隐瞒、缓报、谎报或者授意他人隐瞒、缓报、谎报。

（六）医院感染暴发事件信息通报与发布

1. 经调查核实发生以下情形时，医院应当按《医院感染暴发报告及处置管理规范》的规定由院感组于12小时内向江夏区卫生行政部门和江夏区疾病预防控制中心报告。

（1）5例以上疑似医院感染暴发。

（2）3例以上医院感染暴发。

2. 发生以下情形时，医院应当按照《国家突发公共卫生事件相关信息报告管理工作规范（试行）》的要求，在2小时内向江夏区卫生行政部门报告，并同时向江夏区疾病预防控制机构中心报告。

（1）10例以上的医院感染暴发。

（2）发生特殊病原体或者新发病原体的医院感染。

（3）可能造成重大公共影响或者严重后果的医院感染。

（七）医院感染暴发事件应急反应和终结

1.医院感染暴发的应急反应

（1）当临床科室出现医院感染暴发趋势或确认暴发时立即向医务管理部和院感组报告，院感组专职人员接到通知后，应立刻到达病区，对感染病例进行核查、确认，初步确认暴发后立即报告院领导和各相关部门，启动预案。

（2）医院感染暴发应急领导小组应及时组织相关部门配合院感组开展流行病学调查与感染暴发的控制处置工作，并从人力、物力和财力方面予以保证。

（3）在医院感染暴发应急领导小组的统一安排下，由感染防控应急处理专家负责感染防控救治工作。

（4）院感组在应急领导小组的指导下加强疫情监测，密切注意疫情动态。

（5）医院感染暴发应急领导小组深入做好各项具体工作的检查督导，采取消毒隔离等措施防止疫情的继续扩散。

（6）各业务科室和职能部门要严格做好患者诊治、诊疗场所的消毒隔离和医务人员的个人防护工作。

（7）宣传部门做好卫生宣教工作。

（8）医院财务、设备、药剂部门根据医院感染暴发应急领导小组要求及时提供院内紧急疫情控制所需的经费、物资、药品等紧急支持。

（9）应急反应中相关科室及部门职责：

1）各临床科室职责：

①当科室发现医院感染散发病例时，应及时通过院内医院感染监测信息软件于24小时内完成医院感染散发病例的报告工作，发现医院感染暴发趋势时应立即报告院感组。

②遇可疑病例时应及时邀请感染科医师会诊。

③及时送病原学检查和药敏试验，查找感染源和感染途径，积极治疗患者，控制医院感染的蔓延。

④科室医院感染管理小组及时组织力量查找发生医院感染的原因，及时向院感组报告。

⑤积极协助相关部门完成流行病学调查，认真制定和执行医院感染控制措施，如确诊为传染病的医院感染，按《传染病防治法》和《传染病信息报告管理规范》的要求进行报告。

⑥必要时组织护理人员实施分组护理和限制患者的转入转出。

⑦医院感染患者的安置原则应为：感染患者与非感染患者分开，同类感染患者相对集中，特殊感染患者单独安置，由传染病导致的特殊感染患者须按《传染病防治法》的规定进行处置。

⑧强化手卫生、严格执行消毒措施、进行科室人员的医院感染防控知识和技能的教育和培训等。

2）院感组的职责：

①立即组织专职人员进行流行病学调查，并与临床科室协调配合，认真收集流行病学资料。

②查找感染源：对感染患者、接触者、可疑感染源、环境、物品、医务人员及陪护人员等进行病原学调查，认真收集微生物学资料。

③证实医院感染暴发：对怀疑同期发生的同类感染病例，立即组织感染科专家进行会诊，及时确诊，按《医院感染暴发报告及处置管理规范》的规定证实是否存在医院感染暴发，并向主管院长汇报，同时向医务组、护理组报告并通知药剂科、保洁部门等协助调查。

④与科室讨论制定相应的控制措施。对科室进行感染控制措施指导和督查。

A. 将疑似暴发或暴发患者集中隔离、分组护理并限制探视，并加强医护人员的个人防护。每天用1000mg/L的有效氯消毒液擦拭物体表面3次，即上午、下午、晚上各1次。若将患者集中隔离后暴发仍未控制，则考虑暂停接收新患者等措施。

B. 加强执行手卫生和无菌技术操作。

C. 合理使用抗感染药物，控制某些特殊抗菌药物的应用。

D. 加强可复用诊疗器械的清洁消毒。

E. 保护易感患者，如果医院感染病例是传染病，按照《传染病防治法》相关规定进行管理。

F. 如在流行病学调查和应急处置中遇到疑难问题，应及时向控制专家组咨询和请示。

G. 分析调查资料，对病例的科室分布、人群分布和时间分布进行详尽的描述；分析暴发的原因，推测可能的感染源、感染途径或易感因素，结合实验室检查结果和控制措施的效果做出初步评价。

H. 组织专职人员进行医院感染的病例监测，观察有无新发病例发生，及时进行效果评价。

I. 写出调查报告，总结经验，制定防范措施。

J. 强化宣传教育，组织医护人员进行医院感染知识的培训，提高其监测和执行感控干预措施的能力。

3）医务组的职责：

①发生医院感染暴发趋势时，统筹协调院感组组织相关科室、部门开展医院感染调查与控制工作，根据需要对医师人力资源进行合理调配，组织对患者的及时治疗、善后处理以及对药品和设备的调度。

②当发现医院感染暴发趋势需要对感染病例进行会诊或核实诊断时，由医

教部负责组织相关专家完成病例会诊或核实诊断的任务，并共同制订相关控制措施，指导、监督科室执行。

4）护理组职责：发生医院感染暴发时，根据需要对护理的人力资源进行合理调配，严格执行消毒隔离措施，对医院感染的特殊病例，必要时进行分组护理。

5）感染专家组的职责：

①接受医院的安排积极参与医院感染病例的会诊，指导科室合理使用抗菌药物。

②指导院感组及时完成流行病学调查，并共同拟定控制措施，防范事态的扩展。

6）医院感染委员会的职责：

①及时召开医院感染管理委员会会议，对医院感染暴发趋势进行评估，决定是否启动或终止应急预案。

②及时组织相关部门提供人力、物力、财力等方面支持，及时控制医院感染暴发。

③指导院感组按《医院感染管理办法》的规定上报医院感染暴发情况。

2.医院感染暴发事件终结　医院感染暴发的终结需符合以下条件：医院感染暴发的隐患或相关危险因素消除后或末例医院感染病例发生后无新的病例出现。是否终结由医院感染暴发应急领导小组组织专家论证后决定。

3.医院感染暴发事件后期评估　医院感染暴发事件应急处理结束后，医院感染管理委员会应对突发事件的应急处理进行评估。评估内容主要包括事件概况、现场调查处理概况、患者救治情况、所采取的措施的效果评价、应急处理过程中存在的问题和取得的经验及改进建议。评估报告根据事件分级报告医院领导和／或相关上级部门。

（八）医院感染暴发事件的应急保障

1.人员保障

（1）成立医院感染暴发应急控制专家组：

1）职责：负责对医院感染暴发卫生应急处置进行技术指导；对感染病例实施医疗救治，对下一步预防控制措施提出建议；监督和管理应急处置过程中的安全防护工作，指导开展医院感染暴发事件的流行病学调查；指导医院感染暴发病例的样本采集、运送和病原体检测等工作。

2）人员组成：

组长：一人

副组长：二人

成员：若干

（2）组建医院感染暴发应急医疗队。

（3）根据暴发情况在相关科室抽调主治医师以上的人员组成医院感染暴发事件应急防治队，随时参加暴发事件的救治和疫情的预防控制工作。

2.技术保障相关专业的技术人员的业务培训，应急医疗队定期开展培训和演练，不断提高应急救治水平。

3.物资保障医院设备物资部、药剂科等对应急物资（应急器械、消毒药品、检测试剂、特殊药品等），应有一定的储备基数。

4.资金保障医院感染暴发事件的应急领导小组根据医院实际情况，计划储备一定数额的卫生专项基金。

十六、武汉雷神山医院医疗废物流失、泄露、扩散和意外事故应急方案

（一）目的

为应对我院医疗废物流失、泄露、扩散和意外事故等突发事件，特制定此应急方案。

（二）主要内容

1.本院全体职工若发现医疗废物流失、泄露、扩散和意外事故均有责任立即报告院感组、后勤保障部、医务管理部等监管或主管部门，相关科室应立即组织人力查明原因，并制定防范措施。

2.医疗废物运送过程中若发生医疗废物大量溢出、散落或运送车倾翻、工人受伤等严重事件时，当事人或事故发生科室应立即报告后勤保障部和院感组等相关科室。

3.后勤保障部和院感组等相关科室人员接到电话后应立即赶赴医疗废物泄漏、扩散现场协助当事人或事故发生科室人员一同做好紧急处理措施。

4.由保卫组负责对发生医疗废物泄漏、扩散现场设立隔离区，禁止其他车辆和行人穿过，避免污染物扩散和对行人造成伤害。

5.后勤保障部和院感组等相关科室人员协同当事人员共同确定流失、泄漏、扩散的医疗废物的类别、数量、发生时间、影响范围及严重程度并调查事故原因。

6.后勤保障部相关人员负责对溢出、散落的医疗废物迅速进行收集、清理和消毒处理工作。清理人员在进行清理工作时须穿戴防护服、手套、口罩、靴子等防护装备，清理工作结束后，用具和防护装备均须进行消毒处理。

7.院感组负责指导在被医疗废物污染的区域进行处理时，应当尽可能减少对患者、医务人员、其他现场人员及环境的影响。

8.对感染性废物污染区域进行消毒时，消毒工作从污染最轻区域向污染最严重区域进行，对可能被污染的所有使用过的工具也应当进行消毒，应当尽可能减少对患者、医务人员、其他现场人员及环境的影响。

9.如果在操作中，清理人员的身体（皮肤）不慎受到污染，应就近用水冲洗受污染部位；如不慎受伤，应及时到最近的诊疗室处理。

10.医疗废物暂存点发生医疗废物丢失时，应逐级向后勤保障部和院感组、医院主管领导报告，并尽可能追回丢失的医疗废物。

11.发生医疗废物流失、泄漏、扩散和意外事故时，应按照《医疗废物管理条例》和《医疗卫生机构医疗废物管理办法》的规定采取相应紧急处理措施，并在48小时内向江夏区卫生健康委员会及环境保护局报告。调查处理工作结束后应将处理结果向江夏区卫生健康委员会及环境保护局报告。

12.因医疗废物管理不当导致1人以上死亡或者3人以上健康损害，需要对致病人员提供医疗救护和现场救援的重大事故时，应当在12小时内向江夏区卫生健康委员会及环境保护局报告，并按照《医疗废物管理条例》和《医疗卫生机构医疗废物管理办法》的规定，采取相应紧急处理措施。

13.发生因医疗废物管理不当导致3人以上死亡或者10人以上健康损害，需要对致病人员提供医疗救护和现场救援的重大事故时，应当在2小时内向江夏区卫生健康委员会及环境保护局报告，并按照《医疗废物管理条例》和《医疗卫生机构医疗废物管理办法》的规定，采取相应紧急处理措施。

14.发生医疗废物管理不当导致传染病传播事故，或者有证据证明传染病传播的事故有可能发生时，应当按照《中华人民共和国传染病防治法》及有关规定报告，并采取相应措施。

15.处理工作结束后，院医疗废物管理领导小组应当组织对事件的起因进行调查，并采取有效的防范措施预防类似事件的发生。

16.后勤保障部应加强对保洁公司工人及医疗废物运送工人的教育，加强对医疗废物处理的管理，严防医疗废物流失、泄露、扩散和意外事故的发生。

17.院感组每月检查全院医疗废物管理措施的落实情况，并将检查结果纳入科室的质量考核。

十七、高温防暑应急方案

（一）目的

武汉地区入夏较快，在3月份左右平均气温可以达到24℃左右。疫情期间，雷神山医院工作人员穿戴防护装备，更加加剧了体温的升高，极易出现高温中暑现象。为防止院区人员在高温气候环境下工作出现中暑现象，保证各项医疗工作顺利进行，确保工作人员避免出现或已发生中暑等紧急情况时能迅速有效地启动应急救援、救护工作，最大限度地保障工作人员的身体和生命安全，特制定本方案。

（二）适用范围

本预案适用所有院区工作人员，重点防范人员（各项目管理处）为隔离病室内工作人员、外围支助人员等。

（三）主要内容

1.院感组应在盛夏高温来临之前，提前以各种形式广泛宣传中暑的防治知识，使工作人员掌握防暑降温的基本常识，了解中暑前的身体反应。

2.后勤保障组应加强对各项目管理处在夏季水电供应的管理，保证病区内的用电和用水需要。如遇特殊情况需停电、停水，应事先通知相关部门，并做

好相应的后续工作

3. 后勤保障组应预先采购一批降温药品，按要求将防暑降温物品分发给各病区及各工作小组，亦可根据实际情况再次发放防暑降温饮料。

4. 医务组保健科加强了解医务人员的身体状况，尤其是晕厥、脱水等中暑情况。

5. 院感组与医务组可根据高温情况及病区内医务人员工作情况，采取建议措施：缩短隔离病室工作时间，集中时间进行外围支助工作，预防性饮用防暑饮品，清洁区摆放饮水机等。

6. 轻度中暑者　工作人员在正常工作时出现头晕、乏力、目眩现象时，应立即停止工作，防止出现二次中暑。隔离病区内轻度中暑者，应迅速在其他人员的协助下，在一脱区脱卸防护装备，迅速撤离隔离病室，在清洁区备用凉水、药品、湿毛巾等。

7. 严重中暑者（昏倒、休克、身体严重缺水等）　工作人员出现中暑时，其他同伴应立即将中暑人员转移至阴凉通风区域，观察其症状，以便于医疗人员来临时掌握第一手医治资料。随后通知医务处及院感组，组织救援人员在第一时间将中暑患者转移到最近的医院进行观察、治疗，并上报分管领导。

8. 在遇高温及连续高温天气，有员工发生中暑时，治疗时及治疗后，需多关心员工身体状况，稳定其情绪，告知其安心接受治疗，待体力完全恢复后，可安排再次上岗工作。

第二节 标准操作规程

一、医用一次性外科口罩佩戴流程

实施手卫生

↓

检查医用外科口罩外包装
（需在有效期内且无破损）

↓

将口罩罩住鼻、口及下巴（鼻夹向上）

↓

口罩上方带系于头顶中部

↓

口罩下方带系于颈后

↓

双手食指指尖放在鼻夹上，从中间位置开始，
手指向内按压。禁用一只手指捏鼻夹。
由上至下展开口罩皱褶

↓

逐步向两侧移动，根据鼻梁形状塑造鼻夹

↓

调整系带松紧度

↓

4小时后、口罩潮湿、受到患者血液或
体液污染后，应及时更换

↓

开始工作

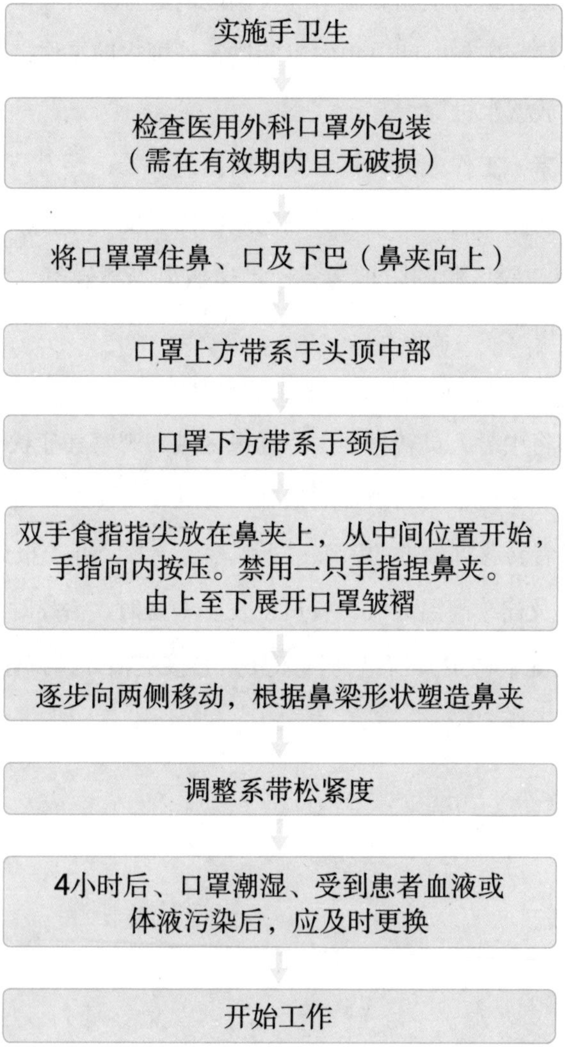

图 3-1 医用一次性外科口罩佩戴流程

二、医用防护口罩佩戴流程

```
                    实施手卫生
```

```
              检查医用外科口罩外包装
             （需在有效期内且无破损）
```

```
               一手托住医用防护口罩
             （有鼻夹的一面向外、向上）
```

```
        将医用防护口罩罩住鼻、口及下巴，紧贴面部
```

```
        用另一只手将下方系带拉过头顶，放在颈部
```

```
              再将上方系带拉至头顶中部
```

```
    双手食指放在金属鼻夹上→从中间位置开始→
    手指向内按压→分别向两侧移动和按压→分别
    向两侧移动和按压→根据鼻梁形状塑造鼻夹
```

```
                 进行密合性检查
        【方法：双手盖住医用防护口罩快速呼吸】
```

```
    若鼻夹附近漏气              若漏气位于四周
```

```
                         调整到不漏气为止
```

图 3-2　医用防护口罩佩戴流程

三、医用一次性外科口罩、医用防护口罩摘除流程

结束工作或者需要更换口罩时

↓

实施手卫生

↓

解开系于颈后的下方系带

↓

解开系于头顶中部的上方系带

↓

用手紧捏住口罩的系带（不能接触口罩前面）

↓

弃置于黄色医疗废物袋内

↓

实施手卫生

图 3-3　医用一次性外科口罩、防护口罩摘除流程

四、隔离区工作人员穿防护用品流程

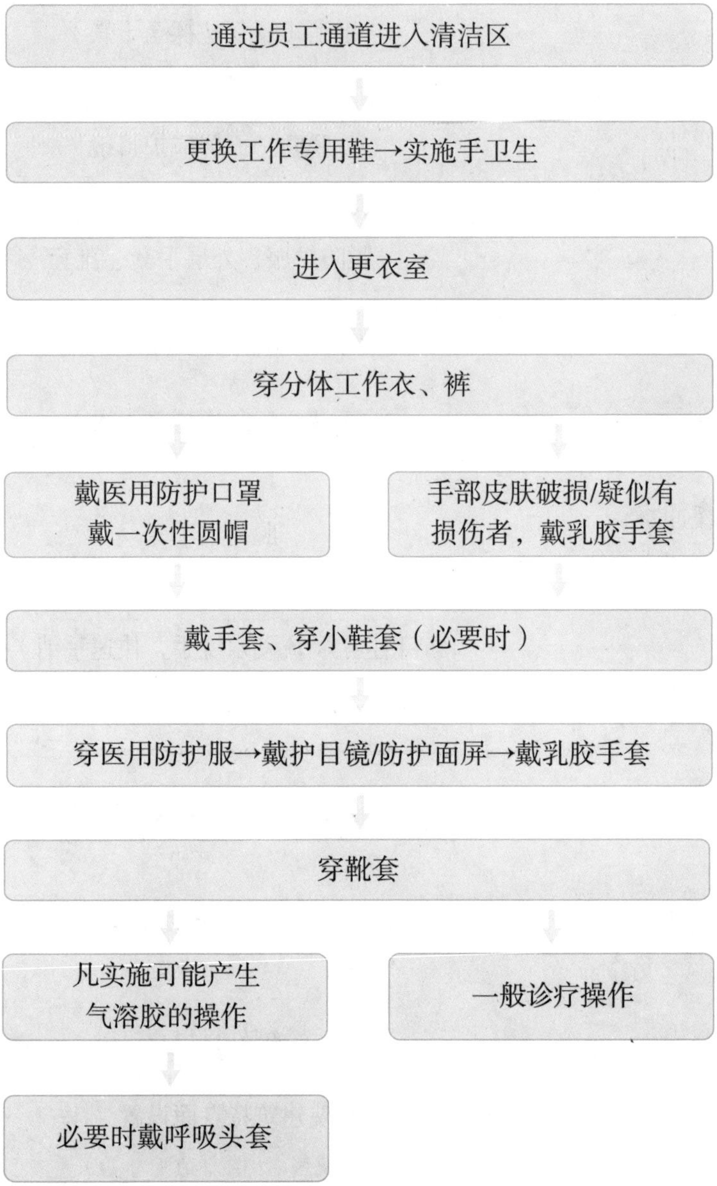

通过员工通道进入清洁区

↓

更换工作专用鞋→实施手卫生

↓

进入更衣室

↓

穿分体工作衣、裤

↓

戴医用防护口罩
戴一次性圆帽　　　　　手部皮肤破损/疑似有
　　　　　　　　　　　损伤者，戴乳胶手套

↓

戴手套、穿小鞋套（必要时）

↓

穿医用防护服→戴护目镜/防护面屏→戴乳胶手套

↓

穿靴套

↓

凡实施可能产生
气溶胶的操作　　　　　一般诊疗操作

↓

必要时戴呼吸头套

图3-4　隔离区工作人员穿防护装备流程

五、隔离区工作人员脱防护用品流程

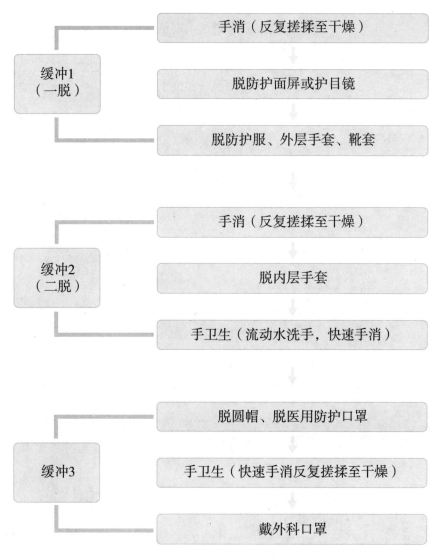

注：以上区域安排根据武汉雷神山医院建筑特点而设置

图 3-5 隔离区工作人员脱防护装备流程

六、工作人员穿戴医用防护服流程

实施手卫生

↓

戴医用防护口罩

↓

佩戴内层圆帽、检查医用防护服外包装 （需在有效期内且无破损）

↓

穿连体防护服

↓

戴好连体帽

↓

拉上拉链，贴好粘条

↓

对镜子进行全身密合性检查

图 3-6 工作人员穿戴医用防护服流程

七、工作人员脱连体医用防护服流程

实施手卫生

将拉链拉到底

脱帽，使其脱离头部，手卫生（分开）

污染面向里，由上向下边脱边卷

丢置于医疗废物容器中

实施手卫生

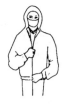 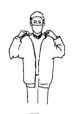 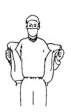 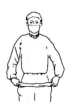 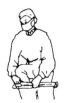

图 3-7　工作人员脱连体医用防护服流程

八、病区清洁消毒流程

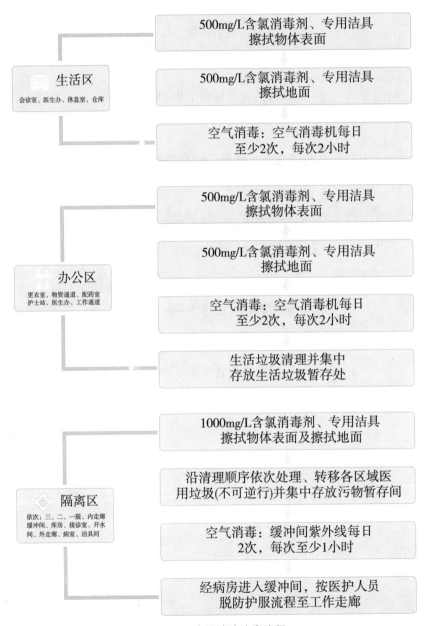

生活区
会诊室、医生办、休息室、仓库

- 500mg/L含氯消毒剂、专用洁具擦拭物体表面
- 500mg/L含氯消毒剂、专用洁具擦拭地面
- 空气消毒：空气消毒机每日至少2次，每次2小时

办公区
更衣室、物资通道、配药室、护士站、医生办、工作通道

- 500mg/L含氯消毒剂、专用洁具擦拭物体表面
- 500mg/L含氯消毒剂、专用洁具擦拭地面
- 空气消毒：空气消毒机每日至少2次，每次2小时
- 生活垃圾清理并集中存放生活垃圾暂存处

隔离区
依次：三、二、一脱、内走廊缓冲间、库房、接诊室、开水间、外走廊、病室、洁具间

- 1000mg/L含氯消毒剂、专用洁具擦拭物体表面及擦拭地面
- 沿清理顺序依次处理、转移各区域医用垃圾(不可逆行)并集中存放污物暂存间
- 空气消毒：缓冲间紫外线每日2次，每次至少1小时
- 经病房进入缓冲间，按医护人员脱防护服流程至工作走廊

图3-8　病区清洁消毒流程

九、床单元终末消毒流程

患者出院

保洁人员穿戴防护用品

拆除床单、被套、枕套等棉质用品

按医疗废物处置，放入黄色垃圾袋内

对全部物体表面及地面进行擦拭消毒、使用床单元消毒机进行床单元消毒

房间无人时，用过氧化氢消毒机进行房间空气消毒

图 3-9　床单元终末消毒流程

十、隔离病区患者外出检查流程

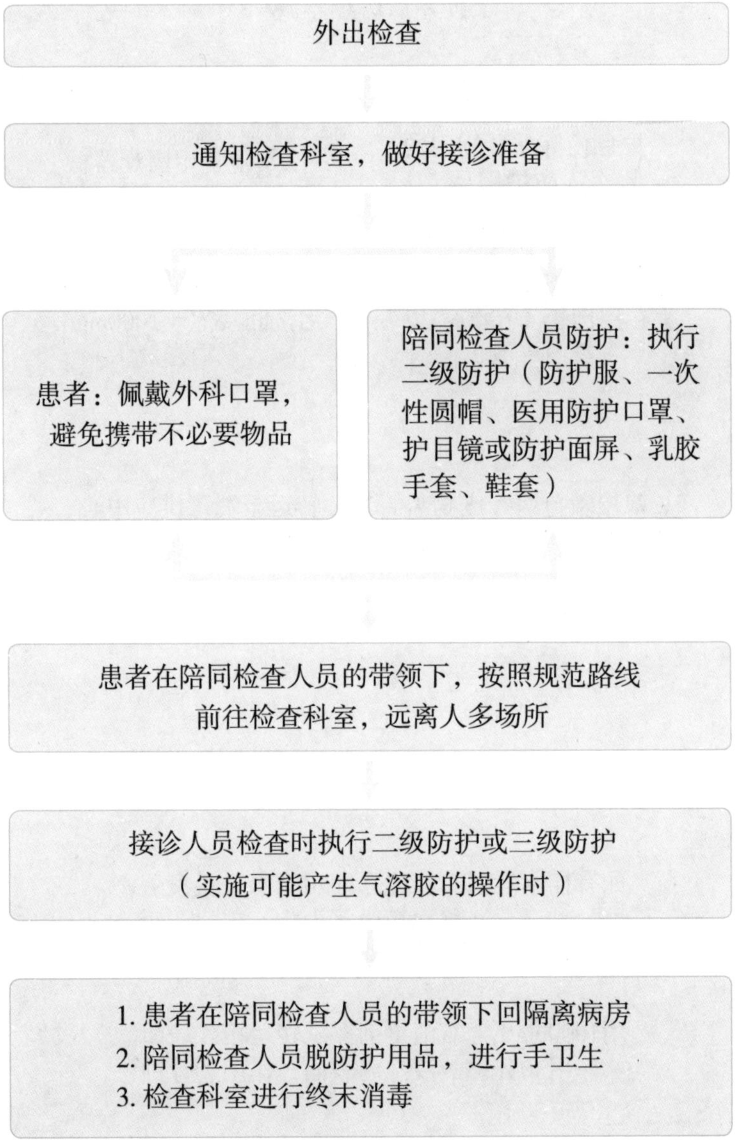

外出检查

通知检查科室，做好接诊准备

患者：佩戴外科口罩，避免携带不必要物品

陪同检查人员防护：执行二级防护（防护服、一次性圆帽、医用防护口罩、护目镜或防护面屏、乳胶手套、鞋套）

患者在陪同检查人员的带领下，按照规范路线前往检查科室，远离人多场所

接诊人员检查时执行二级防护或三级防护（实施可能产生气溶胶的操作时）

1. 患者在陪同检查人员的带领下回隔离病房
2. 陪同检查人员脱防护用品，进行手卫生
3. 检查科室进行终末消毒

图 3-10　隔离区患者外出检查流程

十一、复用医疗器械处理流程

使用后医疗器械

护目镜等需要复用的
个人防护用品

其他复用医疗器械

脱防护用品缓冲间
丢在浸泡箱（1000mg/L
含氯消毒液）

由污染通道转运至
污洗间浸泡（1000mg/L
含氯消毒液）

双层黄色医疗废物袋封装，转运至消毒供应中心

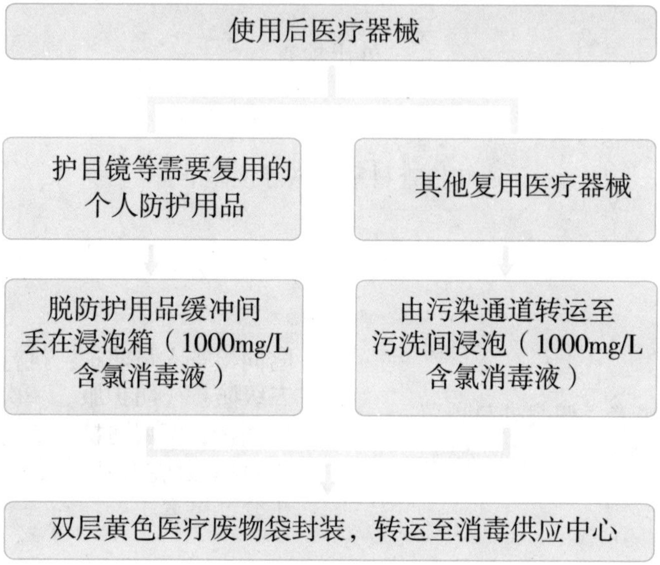

图 3-11　复用医疗器械处理流程

十二、样本转运箱清洁消毒流程

准备消毒物品，做好个人防护

如有样本泄漏时，先立即用吸水材料覆盖，
移除箱内污染物

用1000mg/L含氯消毒剂擦拭转运箱外表面，
作用30分钟，浸泡内表面，作用30分钟

清水擦拭清洁，擦干备用

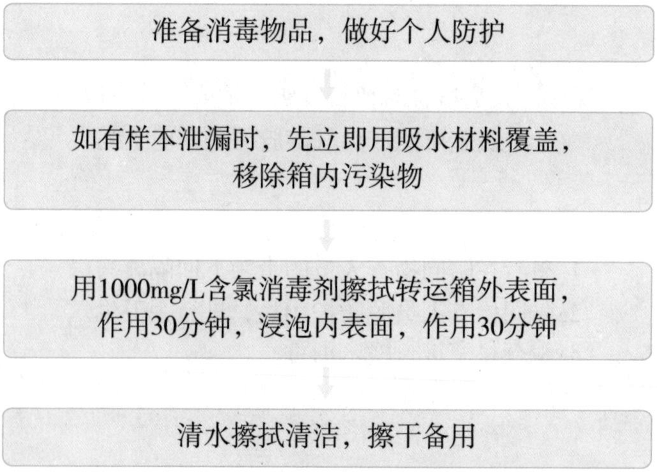

图 3-12　样本转运箱清洁消毒流程

十三、医疗废物收集转运流程图

医院产生的垃圾

生 活 垃 圾
（主要是从行政，医生或护士值班室等洁净区域产生的垃圾）

医 疗 废 物
（主要是从各病区、治疗室、检验科等患者、新冠患者生活垃圾或疑似患者接触过或有可能感染过的区域所产生的废物）

用黑色垃圾袋封装

感染性　病理性　化学性　药物性　损伤性

进行密封打包

分别用黄色垃圾袋封装

锐器盒

送生活垃圾暂存处暂存并做好生活垃圾清运记录

不得超过3/4

送市生活垃圾处理中心

进行密封打包双层包装：鹅颈式分层包扎用扎线带封口
贴标签：包括产生医院及科室、产生日期、类别（标注是新冠）、重量
交接签字：病区与转运人员进行称重交接并双签字留存
出科交接：加套一层黄色垃圾袋或用消毒液喷洒后交接
注意：如包装袋或锐器盒外面被污染时应在外面加一层垃圾袋。严禁挤压袋内防护服等物品，避免产生气溶胶

每次清理完毕及时对垃圾暂存处及运送工具清洗

按指定路线进行转运，且不能和生活垃圾混合运送

送医疗废物暂存处暂存并做好交接记录，尽快运送

送医疗废物焚烧站集中处置，所有交接登记需保存3年

每天运送结束后，对运送工具使用1000mg/L含氯消毒液进行消毒。当运送工具污染时，随时消毒。对医疗废物暂存地的地面使用1000mg/L含氯消毒液消毒，一天2次

图 3-13　医疗废物收集转运流程

十四、消毒液配制流程

做好个人防护（手套+口罩+帽子）

↓

准备相关物品(有刻度的容器，消毒剂和测试纸)

↓

按病区日常清洁消毒制度相关要求浓度进行配制

↓

待完全溶解后用余氯浓度测试纸测有效浓度

图 3-14　消毒液配制流程

十五、新型冠状病毒肺炎患者遗体处置工作流程

患者死亡后，由医院向本级卫生健康行政部门报告

做好个人防护：穿戴工作服、一次性工作帽、一次性手套和长袖加厚乳胶手套、医用一次性防护服、KN95/N95及以上颗粒物防护口罩或医用防护口罩、工作鞋或胶靴、防水靴套、防水围裙或防水隔离衣等

用3000～5000mg/L的含氯消毒剂或0.5%过氧乙酸棉球或纱布填塞患者口、鼻、耳、肛门、气管切开处等所有开放通道或创口；用浸有含氯消毒液的双层布单包裹尸体，装入双层尸体袋中密封，密封后严禁打开

移交殡仪馆

对遗体处置区域进行终末消毒
空气消毒：用3%过氧化氢喷洒
物体表面消毒：用2000mg/L的含氯消毒剂擦拭物表，作用30分钟
污染的衣物等按医疗废物处置

脱下个人防护用品，实施手卫生

图3-15　新型冠状病毒肺炎患者遗体处置工作流程

十六、患者出院感染防控流程

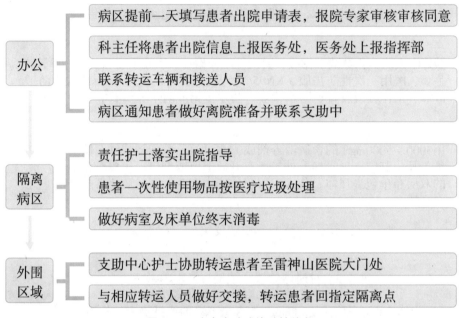

图 3-16 患者出院感染防控流程

十七、防护服破损应急处理流程

隔离区防护服意外破损

迅速用手捏紧防护服周边区域

同时使用胶带，协助密闭破损处

进入"一脱区"，手卫生

脱外层手套，手卫生

防护服破损区域用1000mg/L含氯消毒液喷洒

按照流程，脱防护服，手卫生

防护服破损对应的内层区域
用1000mg/L含氯消毒液喷洒

按照流程，完成脱防护用品流程

重新穿防护用品进入隔离区工作

及时上报感控员和科室主任，扫描二维码
上报职业暴露

图3-17　防护服破损应急处理流程

十八、隔离区出现意识丧失应急处理流程

隔离区工作人员出现意识丧失

↓

第一发现者紧急呼叫支援

↓

将意识丧失者置平卧位，呼叫并观察其股动脉搏动和胸廓起伏

↓

恢复意识	意识未恢复（不能扪及股动脉搏动，无胸廓起伏）
↓	↓
原地平卧休息，测量血压	沿最短路径，抬出隔离区（室外）
↓	↓
症状缓解，缓慢坐/站立，原地观察	解开防护服、医用防护口罩等
↓	↓
在同事陪同下，进入"一脱区"	CPR
↓	↓
按照流程，完成脱防护设备流程	评估职业暴露风险
↓	↓
出"二脱区"，在通风处给予对症处理	进行相应处理

图3-18 隔离区出现意识丧失应急处理流程

十九、隔离区晕厥应急处理流程

出现前驱症状，未快速消失
（如持续的恶心、出汗、胸闷、心悸、便意等）

告知隔离区同事、暂停工作

在相对清洁的区域坐下或平卧休息，酌情吸氧

选择适当PCM动作[1]

测量血压

症状缓解、血压平稳，缓慢站立，原地观察

在同事陪同下，进入"一脱区"

按照流程，完成脱防护设备流程

出"二脱区"，给予相关对症处理

图 3-19　隔离区晕厥应急处理流程

注：[1]：物理反压作用（physical counterp ressure manoeuvre,PCM），包括双腿交叉、下蹲、双手紧握、颈部屈曲等，可升高血压、改善症状并有效预防血管迷走神经性或直立性先兆性晕厥

二十、锐器伤应急处理流程

迅速至缓冲间，脱下双手的两副手套

从近心段向远心端挤出血液至洗手水池

流动水下冲洗

碘伏或75%酒精擦拭消毒

根据伤口大小，酌情包扎

更换新清洁手套

按照流程，完成脱防护用品流程

进入清洁区，重新消毒（碘伏或75%酒精加强消毒），酌情包扎伤口

及时上报感控员和科室主任，扫描二维码上报职业暴露

根据暴露源情况给予预防用药

图 3-20 锐器伤应急处理流程

二十一、双层手套破损应急处理流程

迅速至"一脱区",手卫生

脱下双手的两副手套

手卫生

重新佩戴清洁手套,手卫生

按照流程,完成脱防护用品流程

重新穿防护用品进入隔离区工作

及时上报感控员和科室主任,扫描二维码
上报职业暴露

图 3-21 双层手套破损应急处理流程

二十二、医务人员职业暴露处置流程

双层手套破损	外层防护用品接触皮肤或头发	防护服破损	呼吸道间接暴露
立即到缓冲间脱掉手套		1. 小破损，胶带修复 2. 大破损，立即到缓冲间	立即到缓冲间
1. 用消毒液，如用75%酒精或者0.5%碘伏进行消毒 2. 戴手套	立即就近用含醇手消毒液消毒接触位置	分别到一、二、三脱区按照脱防护用品流程脱去所有防护用品	1. 更换新医用口罩 2. 分别到一、二、三脱区按照脱防护用品流程脱去所有防护用品

报告病区主任/护士长

报告雷神山医院质管院感组

明确下一步处理

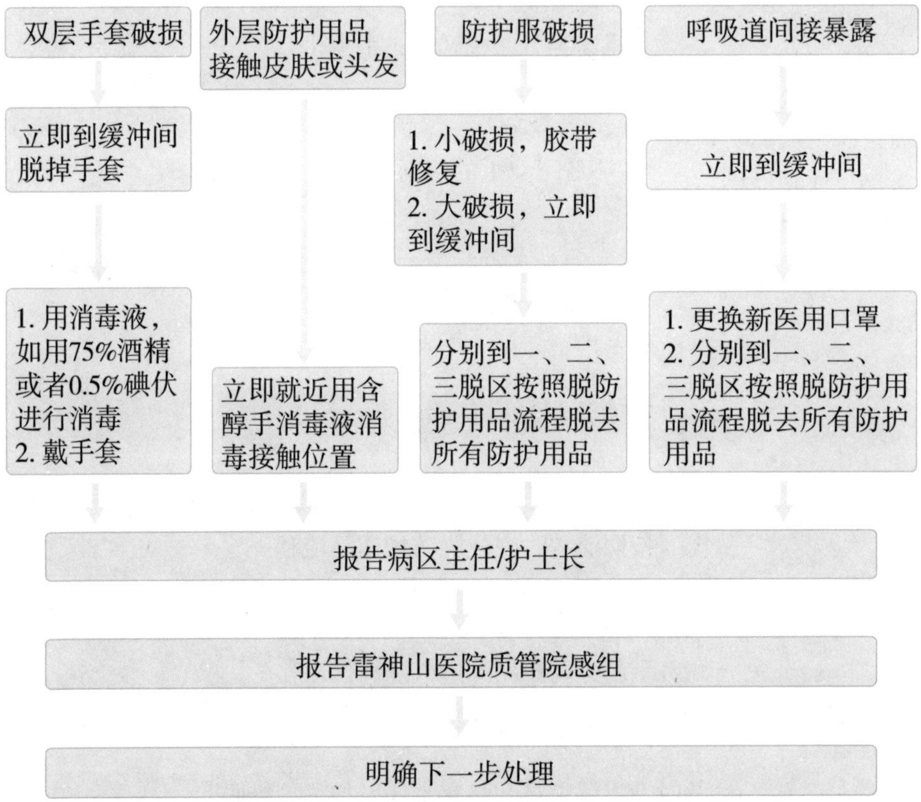

图 3-22　低风险医务人员职业暴露处置流程

二十三、医务人员职业暴露处置流程

皮肤暴露	黏膜暴露	锐器伤	黏膜呼吸道直接暴露
立即到一、二、三脱区脱去污染防护用品	立即到缓冲间	先立即按压、后立即到缓冲间	立即到缓冲间
先用流动水清洗被污染的皮肤后用消毒液，如用75%酒精或者0.5%碘伏进行消毒	1.用生理盐水冲洗被污染的黏膜 2.分别到一、二、三脱区按照脱防护用品流程脱去所有防护用品	1.快速摘双层手套 2.近心端向远心端将伤口周围血液挤出 3.用流动水进行冲洗 4.用75%酒精或者0.5%碘伏进行消毒 5.戴双层手套 6.分别到一、二、三脱区按照脱防护用品流程脱去所有防护用品	1.更新新医用防护口罩 2.分别到一、二、三脱区按照脱防护用品流程脱去所有防护用品

报告病区主任/护士长

报告雷神山医院质管院感组

明确下一步处理

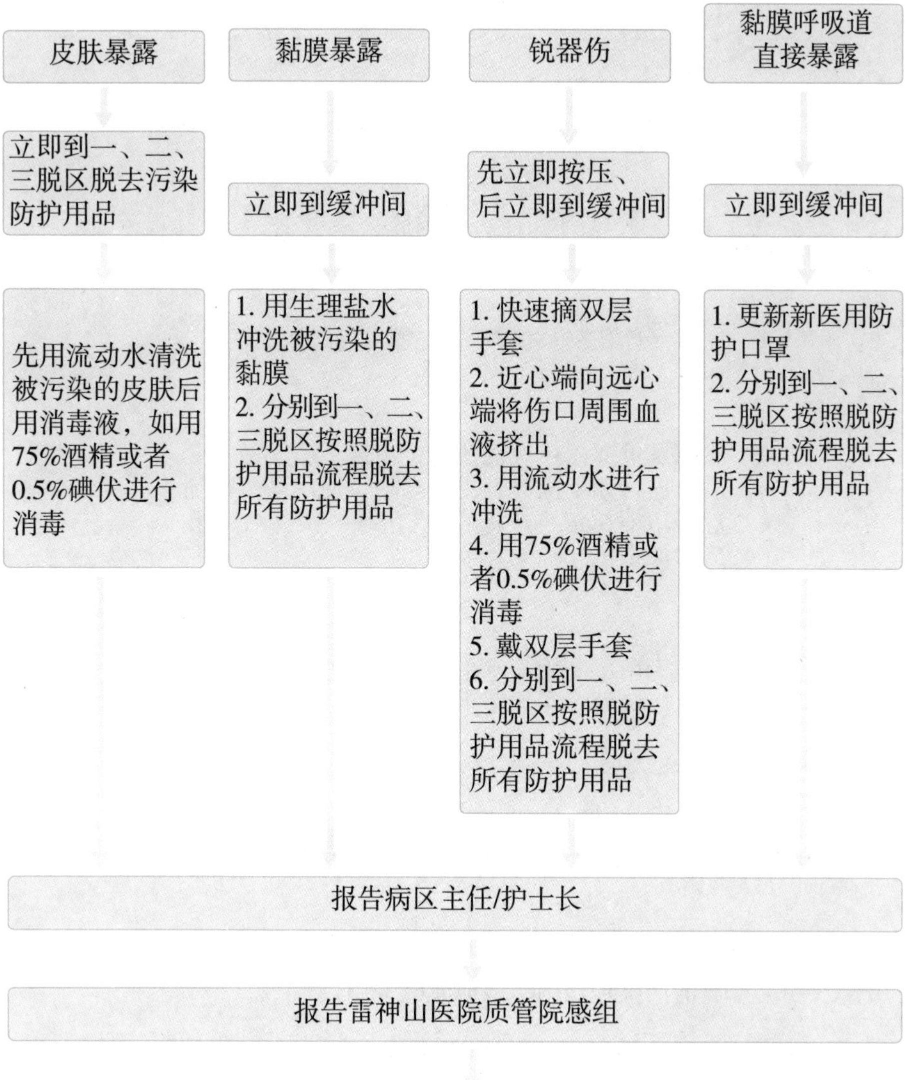

图 3-23　高风险医务人员职业暴露处置流程

二十四、动力送风装置清洗消毒流程

动力送风装置使用后

↓

手卫生，用高水平消毒湿巾擦拭头罩及呼吸管外侧

↓

手卫生，轻柔脱头罩

↓

分离主机，腰带，过滤器与螺纹管

↓

头罩及过滤器一次性使用，更换干净无菌手套后，进行如下操作：主机与腰带使用高水平消毒湿巾擦拭消毒（消毒2次，第一次清洁，第二次消毒）

↓

更换无菌手套用高水平消毒湿巾消毒螺纹管与主机接口处，用无菌手套包裹接口处用胶布密封

↓

螺纹管浸泡消毒后外送消毒供应中心消毒

↓

消毒后的主机与腰带分别用清洁塑料袋密封后放清洁整理箱内，电池充电备用

图3-24 动力送风装置清洗消毒流程

二十五、武汉雷神山医院感染暴发报告、应急处置流程

专职人员前瞻性监测
临床医务人员监测
微生物室人员监测

↓

出现3例及以上相同症候群、相同感染来源及相同暴露因素的医院感染病例

↓

工作时间立即电话报告院感组
下班和节假日报告总值班

↓

院感组到达现场调查、核实 → 确认暴发 → 1小时内报告院领导
医院感染管理委员会

1. 进行流行病学调查，推测可能的传染源、传播途径及感染因素
2. 对感染病例进行病原学检测；对可能的传染源及传播途径进行微生物检测
3. 制定控制措施，初步对感染者、可疑感染者及相关接触者进行隔离
4. 分析调查资料，尽快制定落实针对性的消毒、隔离、治疗措施

本科室医院感染管理小组及其他相关部门密切配合，积极进行调查、分析、控制

医院感染管理委员会启动预案

院外报告：
3例以上暴发或5例以上疑似暴发于12小时内报告；确认5例以上暴发或发生死亡病例或导致3人以上人身损害后果的于2小时内报告；10例以上的医院感染暴发，发生特殊病原体或者新发病原体的医院感染，可能造成重大公共影响或者严重后果的医院感染于2小时内报告

感染控制，预案终止；
写出调查报告、制订下一步防控、治疗措施

报告江夏区卫生行政部门、疾病控制中心

↓

总结经验教训，进行结果反馈

密切配合卫生行政部门进行调查、控制工作：包括调查采样、现场询问、患者隔离、后勤保障等

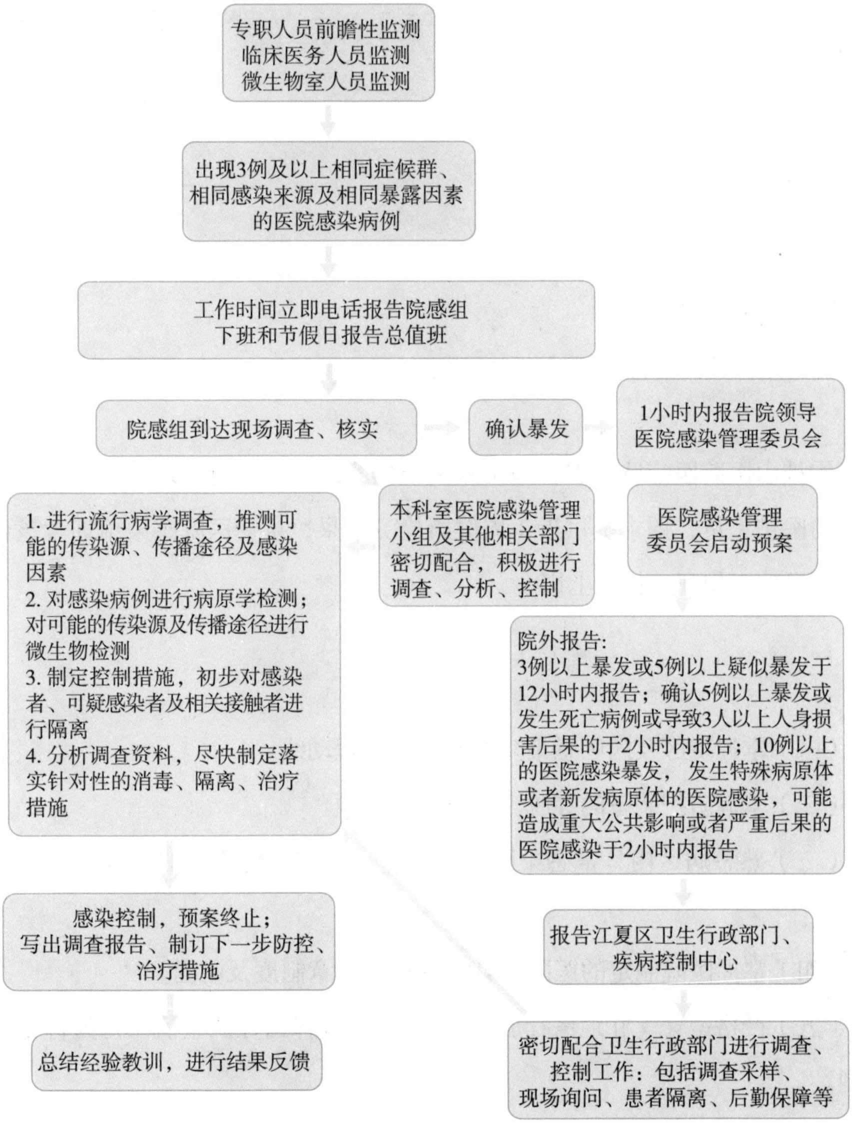

图3-25 雷神山医院感染暴发报告、应急处置流程

（朱小平　茅一萍　王莹　王婷　刘永宁　解莹　翟桂兰　付艳
卢根娣　傅小芳　黄一乐　李敏　张红英　钟倩　赵永娟）

第四章　不同人员的感控指导原则

第一节　医护人员感控指导原则

一、医护人员工作总体要求

雷神山医院医疗队众多，医护人员根据实际情况进行轮班，因此对于入驻病区的医护人员，要求提供近 1 周健康检测结果，接受医院感染培训考核合格后方可发放工作证，持证上岗。

二、医护人员感控指导原则（强制执行原则）

（一）掌握院区及病区感染防控布局及流程动线。

（二）掌握防护装备的穿脱流程及注意事项。

（三）熟悉病区内日常感染防控的工作，并按照院感组的要求认真执行相关制度。

（四）掌握医院制定的医院感染管理相关规章制度及流程。

（五）严格遵守《驻地医疗队管理制度》，确保医疗队生活区行为符合感控原则。

第二节　行政管理人员感控指导原则

一、医院行政管理人员工作总体要求

院区内行政工作人员进驻院区需提供健康证明且接受感控知识培训，相关部门审核后方可发放工作证明，持证上岗。

院区内行政管理人员一律按照工作人员进行管理上下班路程遵循军体路－行政区域。若行政管理人员因工作需要前往隔离病区，应遵守病区入口－医护大街－行政区域开展相应工作。在进入隔离病区前，行政人员应熟悉院区感染防控布局及流程、病区内感染防控布局及流程，并遵守病区感染防控要求，按照病区管理规定规范自己的行为。

二、行政人员感控指导原则（强制执行原则）

（一）掌握院区及病区感染防控布局及流程动线。

（二）掌握防护装备的穿脱流程及注意事项。

（三）掌握医院制定的医院感染管理相关规章制度及流程。

第三节　保洁人员感控指导原则

一、医院保洁人员工作总体要求

院区内保洁人员一律按照工作人员进行管理上下班路程遵循军体路－病区

入口 – 医护大街 – 各个病区开展相应工作。保洁人员应熟悉院区感染防控布局及流程、病区内感染防控布局及流程。保洁人员在院区及病区的活动动线应遵循：清洁 – 潜在污染 – 污染区；污染区 – 潜在污染 – 清洁区动线。禁止随意在各分区随意活动。

所有保洁人员均接受健康体检及感控基础知识的培训合格后方可持证上岗。培训内容包括：清洁消毒方法和流程、医疗废物分类收集制度、职业暴露应急处置流程、手卫生、个人防护装备正确使用等。

二、医院环境地面与物体表面清洁与消毒要求

医院内环境地面与物体表面的消毒一律遵守分区进行。卫生洁具分开使用，清洁区、污染区、洗手间分别设置专用拖布，标记明确，分开清洗，用后消毒，悬挂晾干备用。

（一）清洁区域消毒措施

清洁区地面及物体表面消毒，无明显污染时，采用湿式清洁。当受到明显污染时，先用含氯 500mg/L 消毒液喷洒表面，用吸湿材料去除可见的污染物，然后再清洁和消毒。做到一室 / 区一巾。

推荐每日不少于 2 次（含公共卫生间）。

（二）潜在污染区消毒措施

潜在污染区主要包括病区内的脱 PPE 房间、通向病区内的缓冲间等。潜在污染区建议使用符合浓度要求的一次性消毒湿纸巾，一室一用一丢弃。推荐使用 500 ～ 1000mg/L 含氯消毒液浸泡干巾进行湿式消毒，每日不少于2 次。

（三）污染区

污染区主要是隔离病室、外走道、标本存放间等。污染区推荐使用
1000mg/L 含氯消毒液进行地面及物体表面的湿式消毒，尽量做到一床一巾，
每日不少于 2 次。

当污染区有患者血液、分泌物和呕吐物少量污染物时，可用一次性吸水材
料（如纱布、抹布等）沾取有效氯 5000 ～ 10 000mg/L 的含氯消毒液（或能达
到高水平消毒的消毒湿巾或干巾）小心移除。大量污染物应使用含吸水成分的
消毒粉或漂白粉完全覆盖，或用一次性吸水材料完全覆盖后用足量的
有效氯 5000 ～ 10 000mg/L 的含氯消毒液浇在吸水材料上，作用 30 分钟以上
（或能达到高水平消毒的消毒干巾），小心清除干净。

清除过程中避免接触污染物，清理的污染物按医疗废物集中处置。患者
的分泌物、呕吐物等应有专门容器收集，用有效氯 20 000mg/L 的含氯消毒剂，
按物、药比例 1 ∶ 2 浸泡消毒 2 小时。清除污染物后，应对污染的环境物体表
面进行消毒。盛放污染物的容器可用有效氯 5000mg/L 的含氯消毒剂溶液浸泡
消毒 30 分钟，然后清洗干净。

三、医疗废物处理要求

（一）隔离病区的医疗废物转出隔离区时走专用通道，并在缓冲区再次进
行预消毒或加装包装后交接转运。

（二）每天运送结束后用 1000mg/L 含氯消毒液清洁运送工具。

（三）运送工具被污染时应及时使用含氯 2000mg/L 消毒液消毒；医疗废物
应密封暂存、运输；严禁堆放，防止泼洒泄露。

（四）医疗废物暂存间使用有效氯含量不低于 1000mg/L 消毒液进行预消
毒，增加紫外线光照射不少于 1 小时。

（五）转运与清理人员在进行医疗废物清理时，必须穿防护服、戴手套和口罩、穿靴子等防护装备，清理工作结束后，用具和防护装备均须进行消毒处理。

四、突发应急事件处理要求

（一）如遇医疗废物泄露，应对污染的现场地面用 2000mg/L 的含氯消毒液进行喷洒、擦地消毒和清洁处理，消毒工作从污染最轻区域向污染最严重区域进行，对可能被污染的所有使用过的工具也要进行消毒。

（二）医疗废物转运人员的身体（皮肤）在清理过程中不慎受到伤害，应按照职业暴露的流程进行应急处理。

（三）如遇患者不慎走出其活动区域，应使用有效氯含量不低于 2000mg/L 消毒液对该名患者所有密切接触的场所和器具进行喷洒消毒灭杀。

（四）如遇隔离区发生火情，在火情得到控制后，应使用有效氯含量不低于 2000mg/L 消毒液对灾后现场进行消毒灭杀，并对被疏散患者密切接触的所有场所和器具进行消毒灭杀。

五、保洁人员生活管理原则

院区内工作保洁人员应加强自我管理意识，其员工住宿地应保持干净整洁，经常通风换气，室内要经常进行消毒，如有污染，随即清除和消毒，避免多人聚集。员工若有身体不适症状，按照《健康管理制度》进行上报。

第四节　安保人员感控工作指导原则

一、医院安保人员工作总体要求

院区内安保人员进驻院区需提供健康证明且接受感控知识培训合格后，相关部门审核后方可发放工作证明，持证上岗。

院区内安保人员一律按照工作人员进行管理上下班路程遵循军体路 – 病区入口 – 医护大街 – 各个病区开展相应工作。安保人员应熟悉院区感染防控布局及流程、病区内感染防控布局及流程。一般情况下，安保人员在清洁区的入口和雷神山医院的各主要出入口开展工作，若安保人员需进入病区时，其活动动线应遵循：清洁 – 潜在污染 – 污染区；污染区 – 潜在污染 – 清洁区动线。禁止随意在各分区随意活动。

二、安保人员感控指导原则（强制执行原则）

（一）掌握院区及病区感染防控布局及流程动线。

（二）掌握防护装备的穿脱流程及注意事项。

（三）严格遵守工作职责，做好医务人员出入口、行政工作人员出入口的体温监测工作。

（四）严格遵守工作职责，做好院区内不同工作人员持证上岗的检查工作。

（五）掌握职业暴露应急处置流程、手卫生、个人防护装备正确使用等核心医院感染防控制度及流程。

第五节　维修人员感控工作指导原则

一、医院维修人员工作总体要求

院区内维修人员进驻院区需提供健康证明且接受感控知识培训考核合格后，相关部门审核后方可发放工作证明，持证上岗。

院区内维修人员一律按照工作人员进行管理上下班路程遵循军体路－病区入口－医护大街－各个病区开展相应工作。维修人员应熟悉院区感染防控布局及流程、病区内感染防控布局及流程。维修人员在院区及病区的活动动线应遵循：清洁－潜在污染－污染区；污染区－潜在污染－清洁区动线。禁止随意在各分区随意活动。

二、维修人员感控指导原则（强制执行原则）

（一）掌握院区及病区感染防控布局及流程动线。

（二）掌握防护装备的穿脱流程及注意事项。

（三）推荐在各个病区仪器间留存一套常用维修器械，所带出器械必须带出时，必须经过1000mg/L含氯消毒液浸泡或擦拭消毒，作用30分钟后方可带出。

（四）掌握职业暴露应急处置流程、手卫生、个人防护装备正确使用等核心医院感染防控制度及流程。

第六节 临时工作人员感控工作指导原则

一、医院临时人员工作总体要求

院区内临时工作人员包括但不限于：因公临时访问医院的人员、记者人员、志愿者人员等。临时进入院区人员应佩戴临时工作证，做好登记说明。在院区内的活动动线严格遵守感染防控通道要求，按照其所活动的分区穿戴不同级别的防护装备。

二、临时人员感控指导原则（强制执行原则）

（一）在院区工作人员的带领下按照熟悉院区及病区感染防控布局及流程动线。

（二）在病区感染防控监督员的指导下正确进行防护装备的穿脱流程及注意事项。

（三）需要带入病区的资料、仪器设备等均需提前报备至质管感染防控组，严格遵守病区消毒规范。

（四）需要带出病区的仪器设备等，先使用 1000mg/L 含氯消毒液浸泡或擦拭消毒，作用 30 分钟后方可带出，或使用 75% 的酒精进行擦拭消毒。

（王莹 龚斐）

第五章 工作模式

第一节 病区质控员布点工作模式

布点工作模式是将病区划分为不同感染风险的区域，在每个区域根据感控要求确定督察内容的方法。

一、将病区的风险等级划分为：低度风险区域（清洁区）、中度风险区域（潜在污染区）和高度风险区域（污染区）。

二、低度风险区域是医务人员的休息室。由感控监督员每日至少1次开展手卫生执行和环境消毒检查。

三、中度风险区域是医护办公室和沐浴更衣区。由感控监督员每日至少2次开展手卫生执行、医护人员防护装备使用、使用后织物的处置、拖鞋和环境消毒等检查。

四、高度风险区域是隔离病房、一脱区和二脱区。感控监督员每日至少2次开展手卫生执行、防护装备使用和脱卸流程、医疗废弃物处置、环境消毒等检查。

五、检查遇到的问题及时记录、反馈和整改，并对整改效果进行评价。

第二节　"问题导向式"工作模式

一、"问题导向式"工作模式介绍

问题导向最早起源于课程设计与教学工作，是指教学过程中在教师的启发诱导下，以学生独立自主学习和合作讨论为前提，将所学知识应用于解决实际问题的一种教学形式。目前，问题导向式思维已经广泛应用在各类工作中，是一种日常的、高效的、便于操作的工作模式。

"问题导向式"工作模式的核心思维在于：在树立问题意识的基础上，以解决问题为根本着力点，善于追踪溯源，了解问题的来龙去脉，找到问题的真相本质，探寻解决问题的路径策略。其运行机制应该是：发现问题 – 剖析问题 – 解决问题 – 评价效果四大环节。

二、"问题导向式"工作模式在雷神山医院感控工作的应用

在雷神山医院的感控工作中，其面临着医疗队众多，管理复杂等突出问题，若以常规的工作方式开展工作，在疫情战时期间，工作方式应有所调整。因此，"问题导向式"的工作模式即以发现问题，剖析问题，解决问题为引导思路，可以在一种或一个问题的指引下，不仅可以厘清该类别感控工作的疑难点，更可以进行类似问题医疗队的同质化管理。

（一）发现问题

发现问题首先是问题导向式的第一步。承认问题的主体应该院区内的全体成员，包括医护人员、行政管理人员、后勤支持人员、患者等。在雷神山医院

运行的不同阶段，都由不同阶段的感控问题所在，要善于发现问题。院感组应及时汇总各部门发现的突出问题，集中梳理，例如是否为环境布局问题、流程问题、保障问题等。

（二）剖析问题

院感组对现阶段发现的突出问题进行紧急情况、严重程度进行分类，对急需解决的问题且较为严重的问题，提交医院感染管理委员会进行讨论。在讨论会中，院感组应对如何发现的问题，问题紧急程度，问题严重程度，问题所需协同工作的部门进行逐条剖析。医院感染管理委员会对提交的问题进行解决方案的探讨，并提出各种方案解决的优点与面临的困难点。最终在此次讨论会上应形成该问题的解决方案。

（三）解决问题

由院感组成员对医院感染管理委员会形成的解决方案召开"问题导向式"工作协调会。根据所需解决问题的属性，邀请综合协调组，医务组，护理组，后勤保障组，保安组等多个部门参会。传达医院感染管理委员会的解决方案，并提出解决问题的技术方案与时间限制。在问题解决的过程中，根据情况，可以多次召开协调会，会议的主题即为当前解决问题的进度，发现的问题，需要其他部门的协调解决的问题等至问题解决。在"问题导向式"解决问题常用的工作工具戴明环（PDCA 循环）、甘特图、质量圈（QCC）等质量管理工具。

（四）评价效果

在问题解决后，由院感组向医院感染管理委员会回报问题的解决过程及取得的效果。医院感染管理委员会对其问题解决效果进行专家讨论式评价，并提出下一步工作的重点及思路。

三、案例分享

在雷神山医院刚建设初期，面临着消毒措施落实不到位的问题，院感组了解问题后进行深度调研。以"问题导向式工作模式"为工作思路开展"消毒措施落实"问题解决行动。

（一）发现问题

目前病区反应，消毒措施落实不到位的主要根源在于保洁人员培训不足。梳理细节问题包括方面：新保洁员的岗前培训不到位；手卫生意识不高；个人防护装备使用不熟悉；缺乏正确的保洁流程和方法；对保洁工具的使用不规范等。

（二）剖析问题

院感组在发现问题、厘清问题后，向医院感染管理委员会进行了工作汇报。在汇报会上，达成以下解决问题的主要措施：系统培训（手卫生、防护装备、院区分区、病区分区、消毒剂的配置、保洁流程等）、流程制定（《保洁员工作职责》《保洁员上岗培训制度》《保洁工作流程 SOP》《保洁质量督查表》等）、持续强化培训（制作可视化《保洁工作流程》和《保洁工具分类要求》宣传图）、监督质控（由感控监督员定期对保洁员的日常工作进行督察，督察内容包括但不限于：新型冠状病毒肺炎相关感控知识掌握、清洁不同区域的步骤和流程、防护装备穿脱正确性、不同消毒液的使用及配置、保洁用品使用后的处置等。相关内容可以体现在《保洁质量督查表》中）。

（三）解决问题

院感组召开协调小组会议，根据医院感染管理委员会拟定的解决方案，会同医务组、护理组、后勤保障组、保洁公司主要负责人、病区院感质控员进行方案的分工及解决问题的落实。在解决问题的过程中，随时进行督查，钊对督查过程中发现的问题，由院感组和协同部门共同讨论分析原因，再次制定改进计划，并将改进的方法再次投入使用，观察效果，不断持续质量改进，以保证PDCA循环的良性运行。

（四）评价效果

将问题解决前后手卫生执行情况、防护装备的穿脱正确率、消毒液配制、清洁消毒合格率等结果进行比较。必要时可采用统计学方法，了解持续改进的效果。

第三节　信息化监测工作模式

医院感染防控管理信息系统旨在为医院构建一套完整的信息化感染管理体系，有效预防和控制感染发生，提高医疗质量，保证医疗安全。医院感染防控管理系统依照医院感染防控相关规范、标准、指南，对全院范围患者的感染相关因素进行监控，检索疑似感染病例，及时提供感染暴发预警信息，建立感染报告管理平台，收集并统计分析感染发生情况；建立目标性监测平台，对感染易发患者人群进行过程监测，提高感染防护措施，降低感染率。

雷神山医院感染防控模式之一即是全面实现了信息化监测工作。雷神山医院感染防控信息化监测内容包括以下几个方面。

一、综合监测

基于感染诊断标准、数据标化及经验值，对住院患者感相关染指标做到精准筛查，筛查出疑似感染及高度疑似感染患者，实现感染管理科对全院疑似感染患者的管理，督促临床做好医院感染报卡及感染患者的治疗及防护工作。

二、目标性监测

重点监测感染高发、易发人群，对 ICU、重点手术、多重耐药菌进行专项监测，根据感染指标分析，指导临床做好感染防护。

三、环境卫生学监测

环境卫生学监测对环境卫生监测申请 – 监测 – 结果反馈 – 统计分析等实现了全流程化的管理。便于临床自查，感染管理办公室目标性开展工作。

四、手卫生监测

实现了手卫生依从性调查、手卫生用品维护、手卫生用品消耗登记、手卫生消耗量统计、手卫生依从率等查询统计。注重报表的数据准确性、一致性。此外，雷神山医院特色手卫生监测项目中，嵌入了穿防护装备及脱卸防护装备的手卫生指针。

五、职业暴露监测

根据职业暴露流程，职业暴露要求临床科室上报，方便进行后期的追踪及治疗。

六、穿脱防护装备监测

穿脱防护装备的监测为雷神山医院的特色监测指标，强制要求穿脱正确率为 100%，全面实现电子化监测。此外，雷神山医院在穿脱防护装备检测中，完全实现了电子视频化，即在第一脱防护装备间设置了视频实时监控系统，可由清洁区监控员进行观察，对脱防护装备的工作人员进行语音对讲指导。此外，在监控中，还可以实现手机云端监控（图5-1），高效便捷。

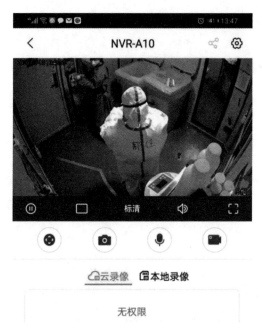

图5-1　脱防护装备云端监控实时图像

（王莹　王鹏　冯毕龙　李锟）

第六章　驻地医疗队管理

第一节　成立感控小组

组建援鄂医疗队后，应立即成立由感控专职人员或感控护士组成的感控小组，在医疗队领队及医疗队长等的领导下，负责医疗队队员的感染防控培训及驻地和医院的感染防控工作。

抵达驻地后，感控小组对驻地和医院进行实地考察，结合实际情况制定驻地感染防控措施，提交医疗队领导小组审核后发布。感控小组还需负责防控措施的落实和督导，包括定期或随机检查，确保措施落地。

第二节　驻地流程管理

一、离开驻地上班流程

（一）穿上内层衣物（无特殊要求，以保暖舒适为宜）。

（二）更换外出衣物和鞋子，佩戴医用外科口罩（随身携带1个医用外科口罩）。

（三）通过电梯离开驻地或进入医院时使用纸巾触碰电梯按钮，或直接触碰后立即使用电梯口含醇速干手消毒剂进行手卫生。

（四）到医院后在医务人员通道的清洁区更衣室脱掉外出衣裤和鞋子，更换工作鞋，再到潜在污染区更换医院工作服，再按流程穿戴防护装备。

二、下班返回驻地流程

（一）在医院脱掉防护装备后佩戴新的医用外科口罩，穿上外出衣裤和鞋子，做手卫生后离开医院。特别注意触碰电梯按钮及其他公共物品后要做手卫生。

（二）抵达驻地门口时先用含醇速干手消毒剂做手卫生，再取下医院戴回的口罩丢弃在驻地门口配备的专用垃圾桶中。

（三）做手卫生后佩戴随身携带的新医用外科口罩。

（四）驻地门口配备体温枪，队员自行测试体温，如有异常及时报告感控小组；测试后进行手卫生再进入驻地。

（五）通过电梯或楼梯返回房间，坐电梯时使用纸巾触碰电梯按钮，或直接触碰后立即使用电梯口含醇速干手消毒剂进行手卫生。

三、进入驻地房间流程

（一）根据驻地房间情况将房间相对划区（图6-1），进门处为非清洁区（注意并非污染区，以免跟医院污染区混淆），浴室为清洗区，房间内部为清洁生活区（包括床、沙发、桌椅等）。

（二）进入自己房间后立即脱下外衣悬挂在衣橱靠近房门一侧（对半分，靠门侧为非清洁区），脱掉外出鞋放在衣橱最下方格子中，换拖鞋，脱掉外裤；若无衣橱，可以叠好收纳在纸箱或篮子中，放在进门的角落；也可将外出衣物悬挂于门外（安装挂钩或衣帽架），鞋子也放于门外。

（三）进入浴室（清洗区）先洗手，再沐浴，注意清洗耳道、鼻腔和眼睛，不推荐常规使用酒精或碘伏等消毒液对鼻腔、口腔和耳道等黏膜进行消毒，一是消毒液可能破坏皮肤黏膜的正常菌群，二是消毒液对黏膜刺激性较强，对人体有害，还可能引起黏膜损伤，反而增加病原体侵袭机会。若遇可疑污染或暴露时，在医院应急处理又未充分，回驻地后皮肤可用0.5%碘伏或酒精或过氧化氢消毒剂擦拭消毒，黏膜可用0.05%碘伏或生理盐水冲洗。戴眼镜者还需注意取下眼镜进行清洗或消毒。如支援的医院清洁区有浴室，且离驻地较远，也可在医院清洁区洗完澡再返回；如驻地较近，且无可疑污染，推荐回驻地房间再沐浴，避免共用浴室。

（四）更换清洁衣裤和鞋子进入清洁生活区。

（五）外出衣裤可放到驻地酒店提供的洗衣机中清洗并烘干（可使用含消毒作用的洗涤液），内层衣物则自行在浴室中清洗，遇可疑污染时首选废弃，需重复使用时可用含有效氯250～500mg/L的消毒剂浸泡消毒30分钟再清洗干净。

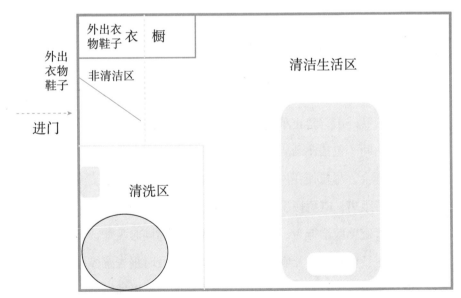

图6-1 援鄂医疗队驻地队员住宿房间分区示意图

四、就餐流程

（一）驻地避免统一聚集就餐，尽量将三餐取回自己房中食用。

（二）取餐须佩戴医用外科口罩（不必戴 N95 口罩），并使用餐厅门口速干手消毒剂严格进行手卫生后再取餐。

（三）避免穿外出服取餐，应穿清洁衣物取餐。

（四）如在驻地餐厅就餐，尽量选择人少时错峰就餐，避免两人对面进餐（间隔 1.5 米以上），避免交谈，取下的口罩内侧折叠后用纸巾包好，避免直接放在餐桌上。

（五）尽量避免在医院就餐，优先回驻地就餐；如需在医院就餐，也应尽量错峰就餐，保持足够距离，避免交谈。

第三节　人员行为管理

一、避免因私会见当地亲友，可通过电话、微信等网络方式联系。

二、避免因私外出，禁止单人出行，确有必要外出须报备领队。

三、离开房间（包括在酒店内部、开会）必须随时佩戴口罩。

四、减少开会，尽量使用网络举行会议；杜绝娱乐性聚会，避免串门；面对面交流时保持距离，避免握手。

五、吸烟者避免散烟行为，杜绝 2 人以上近距离同时吸烟。

六、队员每日监测体温及躯体症状，如有异常及时报告感控小组。

七、队员房中垃圾及时自行提到每层楼楼梯间的垃圾桶倾倒。

八、注意保暖和补充水分，防止感冒，多吃水果和蔬菜，保证良好的睡眠和休息。

九、驻地为每位队员提供单间住宿，不可多人同住，以减小交叉感染风险，并保证休息互不干扰。

第四节 清洁消毒

一、空气净化和消毒

无感染时空气无需专门消毒，每日开门开窗通风 2 ～ 3 次即可，每次 0.5 小时；若驻地为中央空调，如无专业管理人员建议不开启，若为独立空调开启则无影响。

二、地面清洁消毒

武汉驻地一般每日有当地人员统一进行电梯、走廊及各个房间的地面（含氯消毒剂或二氧化氯消毒剂）喷洒消毒，若无统一消毒则可自行使用上述消毒液喷洒或拖拭消毒，注意浓度不宜过高（如含有效氯 500mg/L 即可，过高对呼吸道刺激性较强）；消毒后注意开门窗通风，减少刺激；作用 30 分钟后再使用拖把蘸清水将地面拖拭干净。

三、物体表面清洁消毒

使用可达中高水平的消毒卫生湿巾或 75% 酒精自行擦拭消毒室内物体表面，重点是高频接触的浴室、门把手、开关、桌子、手机、房卡等（不推荐使用含氯消毒剂擦拭，因其腐蚀性较强且需要作用时间也较长）；使用酒精时须注意安全，远离明火。

四、衣物清洁与消毒

衣物需时常清洗；外出衣裤和鞋子不推荐随时喷洒消毒，一是因为消毒液的刺激性可损伤呼吸道黏膜，二是尚无循证医学证据表明衣服和鞋子是病毒的重要传播媒介。而接触了衣物和鞋子的手的清洁消毒才是最重要的环节。

五、手卫生

驻地应在房间及公共区域设置方便取用的含醇速干手消毒剂，比如驻地门口、电梯口、电梯间、餐厅门口等。队员接触公共物品后随时进行手卫生。

六、交通工具清洁消毒

驻地与医院之间距离不宜安排过远，队员到医院工作如需乘坐交通工具，应固定专用；感控小组还需落实交通工具的日常清洁消毒，确保车辆内表面保持清洁，每日可用含氯 500mg/L 的消毒液擦拭消毒 1 次，作用 30 分钟后再用清水擦拭干净，时常开窗通风。

第五节　感染监测和应急处置流程

一、自我体温及躯体症状监测

每名队员每日自我监测体温（如驻地入口处、医院清洁通道入口处）和躯体症状，如有发热（＞37.3℃）或典型症状，如干咳、胸闷、发热、呼吸困难、乏力、腹泻（排除饮食和紧张因素）等，立即报告感控小组。

二、每日健康问卷调查

感控小组制定医疗队每日健康状况调查问卷（建议使用微信），发送到医疗队微信群，每名队员每日自觉如实填写。

三、每日健康评估

医疗队成立由呼吸、传染和重症等医疗专家组成的感染评估专家组。感控小组每日收集队员健康情况，将有症状的队员名单反馈给感染评估专家组，并通知该队员立即返回自己房间进行单间隔离（在单间中休息，避免外出，三餐可由固定人员送到门外使用塑料袋悬挂在门把手上，通知隔离者自取）；由专家组对有症状的队员进行逐一评估。

四、评估处置流程

根据询问危险因素及症状进行风险评估，根据评估进行分层处理：①危险因素：工作中较明确的危险暴露（如口罩脱落暴露口鼻、防护服破损、黏膜暴露、锐器伤和无防护条件下密切接触感染者等）；②典型症状：发热、干咳、胸闷、呼吸困难、乏力、腹泻（排除饮食和紧张因素）等；③其他症状：流涕、打喷嚏、咽喉痛等症状（尤其伴随受凉史）。说明：同时具备上述第①条和第②条考虑高风险，行胸部 CT 检查，影像学高度可疑者，立即联系做核酸检测；只具备上述第②条考虑高风险，暂时观察，若有进一步不适，即行胸部 CT 检查，影像学高度可疑者，立即联系做核酸检测；只具备上述第③条考虑低风险，应密切观察，对症处理并自我单间隔离；解除隔离时间也由专家组根据新型冠状病毒肺炎诊疗方案评估决定。

如有检测阳性者，再由医疗专家组进行评估和进一步处理。感控小组立即开展针对确诊队员的流行病学调查，对与确诊队员有接触者进行风险评估，确定高风险者（如：同一张餐桌同时进餐、未戴口罩 1 米范围内交谈、手接触后未做手卫生、使用共用的未消毒物品等），对其进行单间隔离观察，出现可疑症状立即由专家评估进行进一步检测。

（朱仕超 ）

附　录

附录1　武汉雷神山医院医院感染防控监测指南（第一版）

武汉雷神山医院是收治新型冠状病毒肺炎的定点医院，在特殊时期，及时有效的医院感染防控监测是防止医务人员感染、患者发生其他院内感染的有效措施之一。特殊时期，武汉雷神山医院的医院感染防控监测应当结合医院特色与实际情况，故本监测内容在《医院感染防控管理办法》《医院感染防控监测规范 WS/T312-2009》《医院隔离技术规范 WS/T 311-2009》的要求上融入雷神山医院的特殊情况，特制订《武汉雷神山医院医院感染防控监测内容（第一版）》，供各病区参考使用。

- 强制指标要求全部病区执行，并由病区负责人签字。
- 推荐指标病区根据实际情况进行监测。
- 武汉雷神山医院特殊感染防控监测指标实行日监测，每周向感染防控办进行汇总。
- 其他推荐监测指标按照《医院感染监测规范 WS/T312-2009》进行监测。
- 发现除新型冠状病毒肺炎外的院内感染暴发。
- 强制感染防控监测指标（5个）要求全病区监测
- 推荐监测指标根据情况选择性监测。

一、武汉雷神山医院强制感染防控监测指标

（一）防护装备穿戴合格率（强制要求）

1. 指标要求：100%

2. 计算公式　防护用品穿戴合格率 $= \dfrac{\text{观察防护用品穿戴合格次数}}{\text{观察防护用品穿戴次数}} \times 100\%$

3. 监测操作要求

（1）推荐每日每班由病区内感染防控质控员在防护装备穿戴区监测每位即将进入隔离区内工作人员的防护装备穿戴情况，记录穿戴总人数、正确穿戴人数，并做统计。若病区实有困难时，可以随机抽查检查，每日监测人数不少于当日进入隔离病区人次的60%。

（2）及时发现穿戴不合格医务人员，及时现场给予指导并纠正。

（3）强制要求正确率为100%。

4. 监测记录形式

（1）推荐病区内在办公区、穿戴防护装备区建立穿戴防护装备登记本（根据科室情况自行安排）。

（2）每周各病区向感染防控办进行数据汇总并上报。

（二）防护装备脱卸合格率（强制要求）

1. 指标要求：100%

2. 计算公式　防护用品脱卸合格率 $= \dfrac{\text{观察防护用品脱卸合格次数}}{\text{观察防护用品脱卸次数}} \times 100\%$

3. 监测操作要求

（1）推荐每日每班由病区内感染防控质控员在防护装备脱卸区监测每位即将离开隔离区内工作人员的防护装备脱卸情况（一脱区），记录脱卸总人数、正确脱卸人数，并做统计。若病区实有困难时，可以随机抽查检查，每日监测

人数不少于当日进入隔离病区人次的 60%。

（2）及时发现脱卸不合格医务人员，及时现场给予指导并纠正。

（3）强制要求正确率为 100%。

4. 监测记录形式

（1）推荐病区内在办公区设立脱卸防护装备登记本（根据科室情况自行安排）。

（2）每周各病区向感染防控办进行数据汇总并上报。

（三）手卫生依从性（强制要求）

1. 计算公式　手卫生依从性 = $\dfrac{\text{手卫生执行时机数}}{\text{应执行手卫生时机数}} \times 100\%$

2. 监测操作要求

（1）每日每班由病区内感染防控质控员在整个病区内随机以观察法，观察病区内工作人员手卫生时机并进行依从性的计算。

（2）及时发现手卫生不合格人员，及时现场给予指导并纠正。

3. 监测记录形式

（1）推荐病区内在办公区建立手卫生监测登记表（根据科室情况自行安排）。

（2）每周各病区向感染防控办进行数据汇总并上报。

（四）手卫生正确率（强制要求）

1. 计算公式　手卫生正解率 = $\dfrac{\text{正确执行手卫生时机数}}{\text{执行手卫生时机数}} \times 100\%$

2. 监测操作要求

（1）每日每班由病区内感染防控监测员（监测小组长或护士长）在整个病区内随机以观察法，观察病区内工作人员手卫生正确次数并进行正确率的计算。

（2）及时发现手卫生不合格人员，及时现场给予指导并纠正。

3. 监测记录形式

（1）推荐病区内在办公区建立手卫生监测登记表（根据科室情况自行安排）。

（2）每周各病区向感染防控办进行数据汇总并上报。

（五）除新型冠状病毒肺炎以外的其他医院感染防控暴发监测（强制要求）

监测要求：

（1）临床应高度重视除新型冠状病毒肺炎以外的其他医院感染防控暴发事件。

（2）临床应向感染防控办每日报告散发感染防控病例，如出现 3 例以上综合征的病例，需要 2 小时内电话报告至感染防控办。

（3）下班时间报告医院总值班。

（4）感染防控办需对疑似感染防控暴发病例进行流行病学调查，临床科室应予以配合。

二、武汉雷神山医院推荐医院感染防控监测内容

其他隔离病区根据病区收治患者情况，按照医院感染防控监测规范，选择性的开展全院监测及目标性监测。

（一）监测内容

1. 全院综合性监测：医院感染防控患病率调查。

2. 目标性监测

（1）手术部位监测。

（2）成人 ICU 医院感染防控监测。

（3）细菌耐药性监测。

（二）监测要求

监测内容根据信息化监测工作模式开展。实现信息化监测。

附录2　感染防控质量检查及持续改进记录表

雷神山医院感染防控质量检查及持续改进记录表

部门：		病区：	
检查主题			
	检查内容		
检查情况反馈	存在问题或工作成效		
	改进措施		
检查人员签字：		相关责任人签字：	
		检查日期：	
对存在的问题持续改进情况成效评价（科室或职能部门）			
督查员（科室）签字：		督查人员（职能部门）签字：	
		督查日期：	
注：本表一式两份，检查部门与被检查部门各留一份。			

附录 3　手卫生监测表

手卫生依从性调查明细表

序号	日期	姓名	手卫生指征							结果	
			接触患者前	接触患者/患者周围环境后	无菌操作前	接触体液后	接触周围环境后	穿戴防护装备	脱卸防护装备	依从性	正确性

合计：　依从率：　　　　　　　正确率：　　　　　　　病区负责人签字：

附录 4　雷神山医院院感控督查清单

武汉雷神山医院院感组病区巡查工作表

病区：　　　　　　时间：　　　　　　巡查人：　　　　　　总分：

项目	地点	内容	巡查要点	得分标准	落实	未落实	存在问题	得分
病区院感巡查项目	医护工作大道	病区外走道清洁	1. 走道整洁干净	1分				
			2. 外走道间消防通道双门关闭	2分				
			3. 尽头大门关闭	2分				
		无生活垃圾堆放	1. 无任何垃圾及闲杂物品堆放	2分				
	休息室	人员行为、穿着符合规范	1. 无多人聚集行为	2分				
			2. 穿着外出衣或便衣（禁止穿防护服及隔离衣外出）	2分				
	物资通道	无垃圾堆放，无无关物品堆放	1. 无无关物品堆放	2分				
			2. 有洗手服、护目镜等其他消毒物品交接记录	2分				
			3. 双侧门关闭	2分				

续表

病区：　　　　时间：　　　　巡查人：　　　　总分：

项目	地点	内容	巡查要点	得分标准	落实	未落实	存在问题	得分
病区院感巡查项目	病区清洁区	环境整洁	1. 整体环境整洁，物品摆放有序	2分				
		垃圾分类符合要求	1. 清洁区用黑色垃圾袋，潜在污染区及污染区用黄色医疗废物袋	2分				
		医疗废物的放置符合要求	1. 医疗废物登记本，暂存本	1分				
			2. 双层黄色医疗废物袋密闭收集与转运	2分				
			3. 医疗废物暂存	2分				
			4. 生活垃圾暂存	2分				
		防护装备摆放合适，储存准备合理	1. 防护装备摆放有序且有标识	2分				
		防护穿脱符合要求	1. 防护装备穿脱流程正确	2分				
			2. 穿脱流程上墙	1分				
			3. 穿防护装备间有镜子	1分				
			4. 穿防护装备有监测记录	2分				
		消杀用品储存合理，使用浓度符合要求	1. 消毒用品放置合理	2分				
			2. 消毒液浓度正确	2分				
			3. 消毒频次达到要求	2分				
		办公室整洁、清洁	1. 办公室整洁	2分				

续表

病区：　　　　时间：　　　　巡查人：　　　　总分：

项目	地点	内容	巡查要点	得分标准	落实	未落实	存在问题	得分
病区院感巡查项目	病区清洁区	办公室内人员行为符合规范、手卫生的执行、是否存在戴手套使用电脑、是否防护不当（穿防护服、隔离服在办公室区域工作）	1. 禁止穿着防护服工作	2分				
			2. 禁止戴手套使用电脑	2分				
			3. 随机观察手卫生执行情况	2分				
			4. 禁止在办公室吃饭	2分				
	治疗室	无菌操作的执行	1. 无菌操作流程	2分				
			2. 随机观察手卫生执行情况	2分				
		无菌物品的使用、摆放	1. 无菌物品摆放正确	2分				
		医疗废物的处置	1. 利器盒使用正确	2分				
			2. 黄色医疗废物带，暂存至清洁区小侧门	2分				
		锐器使用规范、是否存在二次分拣的问题	1. 锐器使用规范，无二次分拣	2分				
	缓冲区	护目镜的预处理消毒	1. 护目镜预处理位置正确，浓度（1000mg/L含氯消毒液）正确	2分				
			2. 护目镜转运流程正确，有消毒记录	2分				
		缓冲区的清洁消毒	1. 缓冲区墙面、地面、物体表面消毒记录	2分				

续表

病区：		时间：	巡查人：				总分：	
项目	地点	内容	巡查要点	得分标准	落实	未落实	存在问题	得分
病区院感巡查项目	缓冲区	物品摆放合理	1. 手消摆放	1分				
			2. 镜子摆放	1分				
			3. 垃圾桶摆放	1分				
	病区	环境整洁、无垃圾堆放	1. 环境整洁，医疗废物处理及时	1分				
		保洁人员的工作范围符合病区要求	1. 保洁人员做到：洁污分开，频次达到要求	2分				
		保洁人员消毒液的使用规范	1. 消毒液配备达到标准（浓度测试纸）	2分				
		清洁使用的毛巾、地巾的数量充足，使用规范	1. 毛巾、地巾分区放置使用符合规范	2分				
		保洁人员是否囤积病区纸盒等垃圾	1. 病区暂存间等其他辅助用房无无关物品堆放	2分				
		设备仪器的消毒落实（人员、频次、浓度）	1. 病区仪器设备消毒记录	2分				
		落实医疗废物分类收集（如锐器盒的使用——加盖使用，3/4扎口）	1. 病区医疗废物双层密闭收集，有交接记录	2分				
		落实医疗废物的交接	1. 病区医疗废物双层密闭收集，有交接记录	2分				
		病区负压监测表正常	1. 病区负压表运行正常（5Pa）	1分				

续表

病区：　　　　　　时间：　　　　　　巡查人：　　　　　　总分：

项目	地点	内容	巡查要点	得分标准	落实	未落实	存在问题	得分
病区院感巡查项目	管理	院感质控监测指标完成情况	1. 穿脱防护装备、手卫生等指标监测记录	2分				
		病区医院感染培训情况	1. 病区医院感染培训记录、签到表、培训考核	2分				
		应急预案：科室是否已经培训、人员掌握情况	1. 病区应急预案及知晓情况	2分				
		通道的管理：各个通道人员限制，各个通道规范关闭	1. 各缓冲间门长闭	2分				
			2. 各通道进出门长闭	2分				
		紫外线的使用：计时、消毒、登记	1. 紫外线灯管、空气消毒机使用时间登记	1分				

附录 5 雷神山医院清洁消毒检查表

病区名称： 检查日期： 检查者：

是否有清洁消毒制度	□ 是 □ 否
是否经过岗前培训	□ 是 □ 否
保洁用消毒液的浓度是否符合要求	□ 是 □ 否
保洁工具是否分区、分颜色使用	□ 是 □ 否
清洁使用的毛巾的数量充足	□ 是 □ 否
清洁使用的地巾的数量充足	□ 是 □ 否
隔离病区的每日消毒的频次	□ 1次/日 □ 2次/日 □ 3次及以上/日
保洁工作的内容范围	□ 公共区域地面 □ 病室内地面 □ 公共区域桌面等物体表面 □ 病室内物体表面 □ 床栏、床旁桌等 □ 仪器设备表面
物体表面使用的清洁工具	□ 抹布 □ 一次性湿巾
是否存在清洁工具二次浸泡	□ 是 □ 否
设备仪器是否进行日常清洁消毒	□ 是 □ 否
仪器设备消毒的频次	□ 1次/日 □ 2次/日 □ 3次以上/日

续表

仪器设备消毒使用的消毒剂浓度	□ 含氯消毒剂 　○ 500mg/L 　○ 500 ~ 1000mg/L 　○ 1000 ~ 2000mg/L 　○ 2000mg/L 以上 □ 75% 酒精 □ 消毒湿巾 □ 其他

附录 6 雷神山医院个人防护指引（第一版）

武汉雷神山医院个人防护指引（第一版）

区域		工作形式	医用外科口罩	医用防护口罩	圆帽	手套	护目镜或面屏	洗手服	鞋套	防护服	靴套	隔离衣	工作服	特别说明
非医疗行为区域	办公区、生活区等非医疗区域，包括但不限于办公区、物资仓库、酒店、医务人员入出口处、病区内医护工作大道及其他清洁区域		√							×	×	×	×	
病区外污染走向区域	根据质管院感办所制医院院区感通道示意图，病区外污染走向	患者转运、患者外出检查、标本送检、医疗废物转运生活垃圾转运等人员		√	√	√	√（必要时）			√	√			其区域人员禁止穿着防护用品逆向行走至清洁区，严格按照要求在规定区域穿脱防护用品

续表

区域	工作形式	医用外科口罩	医用防护口罩	圆帽	手套	护目镜或面屏	洗手服	鞋套	防护服	靴套	隔离衣	工作服	特别说明
病区内清洁区 根据质管院感办所制医院院区院感通道示意图，特指各病区内的医生办公室、护士站、治疗室、更衣室等		√	√（必要时）	√			√				√（必要时）	√（必要时）	此区域人员禁止穿着隔离衣及工作服直接及外出至非医疗行为区
病区内潜在污染区及污染区 根据质管院感办所制医院院区院感通道示意图，特指各区病室及外走道等		√（必要时）	√	√	√（双层）	√	√	√（必要时）	√	√	√（必要时）		此区域人员禁止穿着防护用品逆向行走至清洁区，严格按照流程及动线脱卸防护用品后至清洁区域，外出陪同患者检查时，型患者通道进出

注：√为推荐项目，×为禁止项目

附录 7 武汉雷神山医院感染暴发报告的信息核查机制

为进一步提高我院识别和处置医院感染暴发能力，防止其进一步蔓延，保障患者医疗质量以及医务人员的职业安全，特制定本医院感染暴发报告的信息核查机制。

一、核查制度

（一）临床科室患者的主管医生和感控护士发现科室短时间内出现 3 例以上同种病原体感染，且耐药谱高度相同或完全一致经主管医生初步判断是否为医院感染暴发，若"是"或"高度疑似"立即报告科室主任，主任组织人员对上述病例进行核查，再次判断是否为医院感染暴发，若仍然判断为"是"或"高度疑似"，应立即电话报告院感组。

（二）院感组散发病例监测人员、多重耐药菌监测人员以及片区管理人员发现科室出现 3 例以上同种病原体感染的病例，即报告给院感组负责人。

（三）各途径报告医院感染暴发或疑似暴发后，院感组组织流行病学调查人员立即开展核查工作，院感组视情节的严重情况和工作量的大小增补核查人员。

二、核查对象

发生医院感染的患者、患者家属和医务工作人员。

三、核查内容

（一）核实是否为医院感染。

（二）核实发生的医院感染是否为暴发。

（三）核实患者姓名、床号、入院日期、主管医生、是否有感染、是否为医院感染、感染部位、病原体及耐药情况。

（四）核实家属姓名、是否有感染、是否为医院感染、感染部位、病原体及耐药情况。

（五）核实医务工作人员姓名、科室、是否有感染、是否为医院感染、感染部位、病原体及耐药情况。

四、核查方式

（一）系统核对：通过 HIS 系统的院内感染报告系统查询患者信息并通过 LIS 系统查询病原体的耐药情况。

（二）实地核对：到临床科室调查医院感染暴发信息。

五、相关部门的主要职责

（一）临床科室：做好医院感染病例的网络报告和医院感染暴发或疑似暴发的电话报告。

（二）院感组：在医院感染委员会的领导下组织完成医院感染暴发的调查，包括及时在院内感染报告系统中筛查医院感染病例、确定是否为医院感染暴发或疑似暴发、完成病原体的同源性鉴定等，若为暴发及时启动本院医院感染暴发控制应急预案，尽早控制暴发蔓延。

（三）感染医师：负责核实医院感染的诊断。

六、工作要求

感染控制和管理报告系统中筛查是否为医院感染暴发或疑似暴发。

各科室高度重视此项工作，院感组设专人负责，确保相关信息的真实性和可靠性。

附录 8 暴发个案调查表

（疑似）医院感染病例个案调查

A.1 一般情况

A.1.1 患者姓名：　　　　　家长姓名（若是儿童，请填写）：

A.1.2 患者 ID：

A.1.3 性别：　□男　□女

A.1.4 年龄：　　岁（月）

A.2 发现 / 报告情况

A.2.1 发病序号：

A.2.2 发生感染时所在科室：

A.2.3 曾住过科室：

A.2.4 发病日期：　　年　月　日

A.2.5 发现时间：　　年　月　日

A.2.6 感染诊断及部位：

A.3 发病与就诊经过

A.3.1 入院日期：　　年　月　日

A.3.2 可能的感染原因：

A.3.3 原发疾病：

A.4 临床表现

A.4.1 临床症状：

A.4.2 临床体征：

A.4.3 微生物送检结果及日期：

A.5 高危因素及暴露情况

A.5.1 病室环境：　□Ⅰ类　　□Ⅱ类　　□Ⅲ类

A.5.2 医护情况：主管护士　　　　日常护理护士　　　　主管医生

每次接触患者前后洗手或使用快速手消毒剂 □是 □否 医务人员出勤情况

A.5.3 周围患者是否有类似临床症状、体征 □是 □否

A.5.4 患者接触的相关医疗器械：　　　　使用前后□消毒 □灭菌

A.5.5 近期环境抽查结果：空气：　　　　物体表面：　　　　工作人员手：

A.5.6 有无可疑的使用中消毒液：　　　　　　批号：

A.5.7 有无可疑的静脉注射液体：　　　　　　批号：

A.5.8 本组共有患者　例，本患者为第　例，患者感染源可能来自：

□患者自身　□其他患者　□医务人员　□医疗器械　□医院环境　□食物　□药物　□探视者　□陪护者　□感染源不明　□其他

A.5.9 患者易感因素的调查表

手术名称：

急诊：是□　否□

手术日期：

参与手术人员：

手术持续时间：　　小时　　分

手术植入物：有□　无□

手术切口类型：清洁□　清洁—污染□　污染□　感染切口□

麻醉（ASA）评分　Ⅰ级□　Ⅱ级□　Ⅲ级□　Ⅳ级□　Ⅴ级□

麻醉：全麻□　硬膜外麻□　腰麻□

糖尿病□　免疫缺陷□　泌尿道插管□时间（　　）肿瘤□　免疫抑制剂□

动静脉插管□时间（　　）昏迷□ 低蛋白血症□

引流管部位（　　）时间（　　）肝硬化□ WBC ＜ 1.5×10^9/L □

激素及使用方法（　　　　）

放疗□ 化疗□

气管切开：是□ 否□ 时间（　　　　）

上呼吸机：是□ 否□ 时间（　　　　）

哮喘□ 冠心病□ 肾病□ 慢性支气管炎□ 其他慢性肺部疾病□ 其他慢性疾病□

A.6 患者生活习惯、既往健康史

A.6.1 饭前洗手：□每次均洗手 □偶尔洗手 □从不洗手 □其他

A.6.2 本次感染前是否有其他部位感染 □是 □否，感染部位：

A.7 患者发病前抗菌药物应用情况

品种：　　　　药品名称：　　　　天数/使用起止日期

A.8 实验室检查

A.8.1 感染相关指标：血常规：　　；CRP：　　；PCT：　　；其他：

A.8.2 血清学和病原学检测的调查

血清学和病原学检测：标本类型、采样时间、检测项目、检测方法、检测单位、结果。

注：标本类型包括咽拭子、痰、血、尿、粪便、分泌物等与该感染相关的临床标本。

A.9 转归与最终诊断情况

A.9.1 最终诊断：□确诊病例 □疑似病例 □临床诊断病例 □排除：

A.9.2 诊断单位：

A.9.3 转归：□痊愈，出院日期：　月　日 死亡，死亡日期：　月　日 死亡原因：

□其他

A.10 其他需记载事项

可根据实际情况增加或减少个案表内容，例如：若怀疑与麻醉剂、消毒剂有关，应记录麻醉剂、消毒剂的相关信息，以及封存剩余麻醉剂、消毒剂进行检测的后续情况；若怀疑与植入物有关，应记录植入物以及对同批号植入物进行检测的相关信息；若怀疑与消毒供应中心（CSSD）处置有关，则应追溯相关信息等。

A.11 调查单位、人员和时间

A.11.1 调查单位：

A.11.2 调查者签名：

A.11.3 调查时间：　　月　　日——　　月　　日

附录9　医疗机构内新型冠状病毒感染预防与控制技术指南（第一版）

为进一步做好新型冠状病毒感染预防与控制工作，有效降低新型冠状病毒在医疗机构内的传播风险，规范医务人员行为，特制定本技术指南。

一、基本要求

（一）制定应急预案和工作流程。医疗机构应当严格落实《关于进一步加强医疗机构感染预防与控制工作的通知》（国卫办医函〔2019〕480号），根据新型冠状病毒的病原学特点，结合传染源、传播途径、易感人群和诊疗条件等，建立预警机制，制定应急预案和工作流程。

（二）开展全员培训。依据岗位职责确定针对不同人员的培训内容，尤其是对高风险科室如发热门诊、内科门诊、儿科门诊、急诊、ICU和呼吸病房的医务人员要重点培训，使其熟练掌握新型冠状病毒感染的防控知识、方法与技能，做到早发现、早报告、早隔离、早诊断、早治疗、早控制。

（三）做好医务人员防护。医疗机构应当规范消毒、隔离和防护工作，储备质量合格、数量充足的防护物资，如消毒产品和医用外科口罩、医用防护口罩、隔离衣、眼罩等防护用品，确保医务人员个人防护到位。在严格落实标准预防的基础上，强化接触传播、飞沫传播和空气传播的感染防控。正确选择和佩戴口罩、手卫生是感染防控的关键措施。

（四）关注医务人员健康。医疗机构应当合理调配人力资源和班次安排，避免医务人员过度劳累。提供营养膳食，增强医务人员免疫力。针对岗位特点和风险评估结果，开展主动健康监测，包括体温和呼吸系统症状等。采取多种措施，保障医务人员健康地为患者提供医疗服务。

（五）加强感染监测。做好早期预警预报，加强对感染防控工作的监督与指导，发现隐患，及时改进。发现疑似或确诊新型冠状病毒感染的肺炎患者时，应当按照有关要求及时报告，并在 2 小时内上报信息，做好相应处置工作。

（六）做好清洁消毒管理。按照《医院空气净化管理规范》，加强诊疗环境的通风，有条件的医疗机构可进行空气消毒，也可配备循环风空气消毒设备。严格执行《医疗机构消毒技术规范》，做好诊疗环境（空气、物体表面、地面等）、医疗器械、患者用物等的清洁消毒，严格患者呼吸道分泌物、排泄物、呕吐物的处理，严格终末消毒。

（七）加强患者就诊管理。医疗机构应当做好就诊患者的管理，尽量减少患者的拥挤，以减少医院感染的风险。发现疑似或确诊感染新型冠状病毒的患者时，依法采取隔离或者控制传播措施，并按照规定对患者的陪同人员和其他密切接触人员采取医学观察及其他必要的预防措施。不具备救治能力的，及时将患者转诊到具备救治能力的医疗机构诊疗。

（八）加强患者教育。医疗机构应当积极开展就诊患者及其陪同人员的教育，使其了解新型冠状病毒的防护知识，指导其正确洗手、咳嗽礼仪、医学观察和居家隔离等。

（九）加强感染暴发管理。严格落实医疗机构感染预防与控制的各项规章制度，最大限度降低感染暴发的风险。增强敏感性，一旦发生新型冠状病毒感染疑似暴发或暴发后，医疗机构必须按照规定及时报告，并依据相关标准和流程，启动应急预案，配合做好调查处置工作。

（十）加强医疗废物管理。将新型冠状病毒感染确诊或疑似患者产生的医疗废物，纳入感染性医疗废物管理，严格按照《医疗废物管理条例》和《医疗卫生机构医疗废物管理办法》有关规定，进行规范处置。

二、重点部门管理

（一）发热门诊

1. 发热门诊建筑布局和工作流程应当符合《医院隔离技术规范》等有关要求。

2. 留观室或抢救室加强通风；如使用机械通风，应当控制气流方向，由清洁侧流向污染侧。

3. 配备符合要求、数量充足的医务人员防护用品，发热门诊出入口应当设有速干手消毒剂等手卫生设施。

4. 医务人员开展诊疗工作应当执行标准预防。要正确佩戴医用外科口罩或医用防护口罩，戴口罩前和摘口罩后应当进行洗手或手卫生消毒。进出发热门诊和留观病房，严格按照《医务人员穿脱防护用品的流程》（见附件）要求，正确穿脱防护用品。

5. 医务人员应当掌握新型冠状病毒感染的流行病学特点与临床特征，按照诊疗规范进行患者筛查，对疑似或确诊患者立即采取隔离措施并及时报告。

6. 患者转出后按《医疗机构消毒技术规范》进行终末处理。

7. 医疗机构应当为患者及陪同人员提供口罩并指导其正确佩戴。

（二）急诊

1. 落实预检分诊制度，引导发热患者至发热门诊就诊，制定并完善重症患者的转出、救治应急预案并严格执行。

2. 合理设置隔离区域，满足疑似或确诊患者就地隔离和救治的需要。

3. 医务人员严格执行预防措施，做好个人防护和诊疗环境的管理。实施急诊气管插管等感染性职业暴露风险较高的诊疗措施时，应当按照接治确诊患者的要求采取预防措施。

4. 诊疗区域应当保持良好的通风并定时清洁消毒。

5. 采取设置等候区等有效措施，避免人群聚集。

（三）普通病区（房）

1.应当设置应急隔离病室，用于疑似或确诊患者的隔离与救治，建立相关工作制度及流程，备有充足的应对急性呼吸道传染病的消毒和防护用品。

2.病区（房）内发现疑似或确诊患者，启动相关应急预案和工作流程，按规范要求实施及时有效隔离、救治和转诊。

3.疑似或确诊患者宜专人诊疗与护理，限制无关医务人员的出入，原则上不探视；有条件的可以安置在负压病房。

4.不具备救治条件的非定点医院，应当及时转到有隔离和救治能力的定点医院。等候转诊期间对患者采取有效的隔离和救治措施。

5.患者转出后按《医疗机构消毒技术规范》对其接触环境进行终末处理。

（四）收治疑似或确诊新型冠状病毒感染的肺炎患者的病区（房）

1.建筑布局和工作流程应当符合《医院隔离技术规范》等有关要求，并配备符合要求、数量合适的医务人员防护用品。设置负压病区（房）的医疗机构应当按相关要求实施规范管理。

2.对疑似或确诊患者应当及时采取隔离措施，疑似患者和确诊患者应当分开安置；疑似患者进行单间隔离，经病原学确诊的患者可以同室安置。

3.在实施标准预防的基础上，采取接触隔离、飞沫隔离和空气隔离等措施。具体措施包括：

（1）进出隔离病房，应当严格执行《医院隔离技术规范》《医务人员穿脱防护用品的流程》，正确实施手卫生及穿脱防护用品。

（2）应当制定医务人员穿脱防护用品的流程；制作流程图和配置穿衣镜。配备熟练感染防控技术的人员督导医务人员防护用品的穿脱，防止污染。

（3）用于诊疗疑似或确诊患者的听诊器、体温计、血压计等医疗器具及护理物品应当专人专用。若条件有限，不能保障医疗器具专人专用时，每次使用后应当进行规范的清洁和消毒。

4.重症患者应当收治在重症监护病房或者具备监护和抢救条件的病室，收治重症患者的监护病房或者具备监护和抢救条件的病室不得收治其他患者。

5.严格探视制度，原则上不设陪护。若患者病情危重等特殊情况必须探视的，探视者必须严格按照规定做好个人防护。

6.按照《医院空气净化管理规范》规定，进行空气净化。

三、医务人员防护

（一）医疗机构和医务人员应当强化标准预防措施的落实，做好诊区、病区（房）的通风管理，严格落实《医务人员手卫生规范》要求，佩戴医用外科口罩/医用防护口罩，必要时戴乳胶手套。

（二）采取飞沫隔离、接触隔离和空气隔离防护措施，根据不同情形，做到以下防护。

1.接触患者的血液、体液、分泌物、排泄物、呕吐物及污染物品时：戴清洁手套，脱手套后洗手。

2.可能受到患者血液、体液、分泌物等喷溅时：戴医用防护口罩、护目镜、穿防渗隔离衣。

3.为疑似患者或确诊患者实施可能产生气溶胶的操作（如气管插管、无创通气、气管切开，心肺复苏，插管前手动通气和支气管镜检查等）时：

（1）采取空气隔离措施。

（2）佩戴医用防护口罩，并进行密闭性能检测。

（3）眼部防护（如护目镜或面罩）。

（4）穿防体液渗入的长袖隔离衣，戴手套。

（5）操作应当在通风良好的房间内进行。

（6）房间中人数限制在患者所需护理和支持的最低数量。

（三）医务人员使用的防护用品应当符合国家有关标准。

（四）医用外科口罩、医用防护口罩、护目镜、隔离衣等防护用品被患者血液、体液、分泌物等污染时应当及时更换。

（五）正确使用防护用品，戴手套前应当洗手，脱去手套或隔离服后应当立即流动水洗手。

（六）严格执行锐器伤防范措施。

（七）每位患者用后的医疗器械、器具应当按照《医疗机构消毒技术规范》要求进行清洁与消毒。

四、加强患者管理

（一）对疑似或确诊患者及时进行隔离，并按照指定规范路线由专人引导进入隔离区。

（二）患者进入病区前更换患者服，个人物品及换下的衣服集中消毒处理后，存放于指定地点由医疗机构统一保管。

（三）指导患者正确选择、佩戴口罩，正确实施咳嗽礼仪和手卫生。

（四）加强对患者探视或陪护人员的管理。

（五）对被隔离的患者，原则上其活动限制在隔离病房内，减少患者的移动和转换病房，若确需离开隔离病房或隔离区域时，应当采取相应措施如佩戴医用外科口罩，防止患者对其他患者和环境造成污染。

（六）疑似或确诊患者出院、转院时，应当更换干净衣服后方可离开，按《医疗机构消毒技术规范》对其接触环境进行终末消毒。

（七）疑似或确诊患者死亡的，对尸体应当及时进行处理。处理方法为：用 3000mg/L 的含氯消毒剂或 0.5% 过氧乙酸棉球或纱布填塞患者口、鼻、耳、肛门等所有开放通道；用双层布单包裹尸体，装入双层尸体袋中，由专用车辆直接送至指定地点火化。患者住院期间使用的个人物品经消毒后方可随患者或家属带回家。

附件

医务人员穿脱防护用品的流程

一、医务人员进入隔离病区穿戴防护用品程序

（一）医务人员通过员工专用通道进入清洁区，认真洗手后依次戴医用防护口罩、一次性帽子或布帽、换工作鞋袜，有条件的可以更换刷手衣裤。

（二）在进入潜在污染区前穿工作服，手部皮肤有破损或疑似有损伤者戴手套进入潜在污染区。

（三）在进入污染区前，脱工作服换穿防护服或者隔离衣，加戴一次性帽子和一次性医用外科口罩（共穿戴两层帽子、口罩）、防护眼镜、手套、鞋套。

二、医务人员离开隔离病区脱摘防护用品程序

（一）医务人员离开污染区前，应当先消毒双手，依次脱摘防护眼镜、外层一次性医用外科口罩和外层一次性帽子、防护服或者隔离衣、鞋套、手套等物品，分置于专用容器中，再次消毒手，进入潜在污染区，换穿工作服。

（二）离开潜在污染区进入清洁区前，先洗手与手消毒，脱工作服，洗手和手消毒。

（三）离开清洁区前，洗手与手消毒，摘去里层一次性帽子或布帽、里层医用防护口罩，沐浴更衣，并进行口腔、鼻腔及外耳道的清洁。

（四）每次接触患者后立即进行手的清洗和消毒。

（五）一次性医用外科口罩、医用防护口罩、防护服或者隔离衣等防护用品被患者血液、体液、分泌物等污染时应当立即更换。

（六）下班前应当进行个人卫生处置，并注意呼吸道与黏膜的防护。

（国家卫生健康委办公厅）

附录 10 新型冠状病毒感染的肺炎防控中常见医用防护用品使用范围指引（试行）

一、外科口罩：预检分诊、发热门诊及全院诊疗区域应当使用，需正确佩戴。污染或潮湿时随时更换。

二、医用防护口罩：原则上在发热门诊、隔离留观病区（房）、隔离病区（房）和隔离重症监护病区（房）等区域，以及进行采集呼吸道标本、气管插管、气管切开、无创通气、吸痰等可能产生气溶胶的操作时使用。一般 4 小时更换，污染或潮湿时随时更换。其他区域和在其他区域的诊疗操作，原则上不使用。

三、乳胶检查手套：在预检分诊、发热门诊、隔离留观病区（房）、隔离病区（房）和隔离重症监护病区（房）等区域使用，但需正确穿戴和脱摘，注意及时更换手套。禁止戴手套离开诊疗区域。戴手套不能取代手卫生。

四、速干手消毒剂：医务人员诊疗操作过程中，手部未见明显污染物时使用，全院均应当使用。预检分诊、发热门诊、隔离留观病区（房）、隔离病区（房）和隔离重症监护病区（房）必须配备使用。

五、护目镜：在隔离留观病区（房）、隔离病区（房）和隔离重症监护病区（房）等区域，以及采集呼吸道标本、气管插管、气管切开、无创通气、吸痰等可能出现血液、体液和分泌物等喷溅操作时使用。禁止戴着护目镜离开上述区域。如护目镜为可重复使用的，应当消毒后再复用。其他区域和在其他区域的诊疗操作原则上不使用护目镜。

六、防护面罩/防护面屏：诊疗操作中可能发生血液、体液和分泌物等喷溅时使用。如为可重复使用的，使用后应当消毒方可再用；如为一次性使用的，不得重复使用。护目镜和防护面罩／防护面屏不需要同时使用。禁止戴着防护面罩／防护面屏离开诊疗区域。

七、隔离衣：预检分诊、发热门诊使用普通隔离衣，隔离留观病区（房）、隔离病区（房）和隔离重症监护病区（房）使用防渗一次性隔离衣，其他科室或区域根据是否接触患者使用。一次性隔离衣不得重复使用。如使用可复用的隔离衣，使用后按规定消毒后方可再用。禁止穿着隔离衣离开上述区域。

八、防护服：隔离留观病区（房）、隔离病区（房）和隔离重症监护病区（房）使用。防护服不得重复使用。禁止戴着医用防护口罩和穿着防护服离开上述区域。其他区域和在其他区域的诊疗操作原则上不使用防护服。

其他人员如物业保洁人员、保安人员等需进入相关区域时，按相关区域防护要求使用防护用品，并正确穿戴和脱摘。

（国家卫生健康委办公厅）

附录 11　新冠肺炎疫情期间医务人员防护技术指南（试行）

根据《中华人民共和国传染病防治法》《医院感染管理办法》《医疗机构内新型冠状病毒感染预防与控制技术指南（第一版）》《新型冠状病毒感染的肺炎防控中常见医用防护用品使用范围指引（试行）》等法律法规及文件要求，为降低医务人员感染风险，更好地服务患者，特制定本指南。

一、相关概念

（一）院内感染。指患者在医疗机构内获得的感染，包括在住院期间发生的感染和在院内获得、出院后发生的感染，但不包括入院前已开始或者入院时已处于潜伏期的感染。医疗机构工作人员在院内获得的感染也属于院内感染。

（二）医源性感染。指在医疗服务过程中，因病原体传播引起的感染。

（三）医务人员职业暴露。指医务人员在从事诊疗、护理活动过程中接触有毒、有害物质或传染病病原体从而引起伤害健康或危及生命的一类职业暴露。

（四）医务人员院内感染。指医务人员在从事诊疗、护理等工作过程中获得的各种病原微生物感染，如细菌、真菌、病毒等致病微生物感染。

（五）院内感染暴发。指在医疗机构或其科室的患者中，短时间内发生 3 例及以上同种同源感染病例的现象。

（六）疑似院内感染暴发。指在医疗机构或其科室的患者中，短时间内出现 3 例及以上临床综合征相似、怀疑有共同感染源的感染病例；或者 3 例及以上怀疑有共同感染源或感染途径的感染病例的现象。

（七）院内感染聚集。指在医疗机构或某科室的患者中，短时间内发生院内感染病例增多，并超过历年散发发病率水平的现象。

二、传播途径

经呼吸道飞沫和密切接触传播是新冠肺炎主要的传播途径。在相对封闭的环境中长时间暴露于高浓度气溶胶情况下存在经气溶胶传播的可能。

三、标准预防

标准预防是预防与控制院内感染需普遍遵守的重要原则之，其目的在于降低已知或未知病原体感染传播的风险。标准预防是指医疗机构所有患者和医务人员采取的一系列防护措施，要求医务人员必须知晓所有患者的体内物质均可能具有传染性，需进行相应的隔离和防护。倡导医务人员无论身在何地，进行何种诊疗或操作，只要接触患者，均可能存在感染源暴露风险，均应采取相应的防护措施。

（一）相关概念

1.标准预防　针对所有患者和医务人员采取的一组预防感染的措施。具体措施包括手卫生、根据预期可能发生的暴露风险选用防护服、口罩、手套、护目镜、防护面屏、安全注射装置、安全注射、被动和主动免疫及环境清洁等。

2.个人防护装备（PPE）　用于保护医务人员避免接触感染性因子的各种屏障。包括口罩、手套、护目镜、防护面屏、防水围裙、隔离衣、防护服和个人防护装备等。

3.隔离技术　采用适宜的技术、方法，防止病原体传播给他人的方法。包括空间隔离、屏障隔离、个人防护装备（PPE）的使用、污染控制技术如清洁、消毒、灭菌、手卫生、环境管理等。

4.屏障隔离　是在易感者与暴露源之间采用物理性屏障的隔离措施（如墙体、隔断、隔帘、薄膜）的统称。

5.空间隔离　利用距离与空间将易感者与暴露源进行分隔的措施，如隔离房间。

6.额外预防　在标准预防措施的基础上，针对特定情况的暴露风险和传播途径所采取的补充和额外的预防措施。如呼吸道隔离、消化道隔离、血液体液隔离、咳嗽礼仪等措施。

7.安全注射　对接受注射者做到无害，使实施注射操作的医务人员不暴露于可避免的危险，注射后的废弃物不对环境和他人造成危害。

8.安全注射装置　用于抽取动静脉血液、其他体液或注射药物的无针或有针的装置，通过内在的设计使其在使用后能屏蔽锐器，降低职业暴露感染的风险。

（二）标准预防的原则

1.既要防止呼吸道疾病传播，也要防止非呼吸道疾病传播。

2.既要保护医务人员，也要保护患者。

3.根据疾病传播特点采取相应的隔离措施。

4.所有医疗机构均应普遍遵循标准预防原则，标准预防措施应覆盖诊疗活动的全过程。标准预防的措施不只限于有传染病的患者和传染病医院或感染性疾病科的医务人员。感染性疾病具有潜伏期、窗口期和隐匿性感染的特点，大多数感染性疾病在出现临床症状前就已经具有传染性，因此，不应只在疾病明确诊断后才采取隔离防护措施，而应覆盖诊疗活动的全过程。

（三）标准预防管理要求

1.防护准备　医务人员在从事医疗活动前均应树立标准预防的理念，掌握标准预防的具体措施、应用原则和技术要求。

医疗机构除了做好环境设置和管理，还应为医务人员提供充足、符合标准、能应对各种暴露风险所需要的防护用品（如医用防护口罩、护目镜、防护面屏、手套、隔离衣、鞋套、靴套等），具体要求如下：

（1）在医务人员频繁操作的医疗活动场所和出入口均应设置流动水洗手池、非手触式水龙头，配备手消毒剂和干手纸巾等手卫生设施。

（2）在高风险病区、隔离病区或传染病区应设有专门的防护更衣区域。

（3）防护更衣区城除了配备上述防护用品外，还应设置穿衣镜、靠椅（靠凳）、污衣袋、医疗废物桶以及沐浴设施等。

（4）所有防护用品均应符合国家相关标准，按不同型号进行配备，并便于取用。

（5）防护更衣区的出入口张贴防护服的穿、脱流程图。

（6）制订更衣区域的清洁消毒制度与流程，明确岗位职责。

2.手卫生管理　诊疗活动中医务人员的手是直接或间接接触患者的重要环节之一，医务人员的手卫生是标准预防措施中的重中之重。医疗机构应将医务人员手卫生纳入医疗安全管理，并将手卫生规范、知识、技术纳入医务人员培训中。所有医务人员在诊疗活动中除了遵循《医务人员手卫生规范》外，还应特别强调"一旦可疑接触了血液、体液、分泌物、排泄物等物质以及被其污染的物品后应当立即洗手或手消毒"。

进行高风险操作或无菌操作时应戴手套，改变操作部位或目的时应及时更换手套，脱去手套后应立即进行手卫生。

尽管不同类型的医疗机构、不同专业、不同岗位的诊疗工作不尽相同，但手卫生的时机还应强调如下环节：

（1）下列情况之时：抵达工作场所。

（2）下列情况之前：直接接触患者、戴手套进行临床操作、药品准备、接触、摆放食物或协助患者进食、离开工作场所。

（3）下列情况之间：对同一患者进行不同部位的操作。

（4）下列情况之后：取下手套或取下个人防护用品；接触血液、体液、分泌物、排泄物和被其污染的物品；接触已知或可疑被血液、体液或渗出液污染的物品；无论是戴手套，只要有个人躯体需求时，如使用厕所、擦拭或擤鼻涕等。

医务人员应接受系统的职业防护培训，养成良好的手卫生习惯，将接触传播的风险降到最低。

四、额外预防

额外预防的理念是在标准预防的基础上，结合医务人员操作中可能暴露的风险强度和情形，从安全需求的角度而提出的一种防护方法。

（一）额外预防原则

1.安全、有效、科学、方便、经济的原则，采取按需配备和分级防护。

2.所有人员必须遵循公众意识。

3.面向所有医务人员，所有人员必须参加培训、考核。

4.防护措施始于诊疗之前而不是诊断明确之后。

5.违规必纠。

（二）额外预防的方法

1.基本防护　每位医务人员必须遵守的基本措施。

适用对象：诊疗工作中所有医务人员（无论是否有传染病流行）。

防护配备：医用口罩、工作服、工作鞋、工作帽。

防护要求：遵循标准预防的理念；洗手和手消毒。

2. 加强防护　在基本防护的基础上，根据感染暴露的风险加强防护措施。

防护对象：可能接触患者血液、体液或接触血液体液污染的物品或环境表面的医、药、护、技、工勤等人员；进入传染病区域、留观室、病区的医务人员（传染病流行期）；转运传染病患者的医务人员、实验室的技术人员和其他辅助人员、工勤人员或司机等。

防护配备：医用手套、医用外科口罩、医用防护口罩、护目镜、防护面屏、防护服、隔离服、鞋套和靴套等。

3. 严密防护　由于感染风险特别严重，在加强防护的基础上额外增加更为严密的措施。

防护对象：为甲类传染病、新发再发传染病或原因不明的传染病患者进行如气管切开、气管插管、吸痰等有创操作时；为传染病患者进行尸检时。

防护要求：在加强防护的基础上，增加使用全面型防护器等有效的防护用品。

总之，额外预防对医务人员而言，在标准预防理念下，基于临床诊疗操作中不同的暴露风险，根据安全防护的需要而采取的一种适当、安全的防护方法。

五、医务人员穿脱防护用品流程

参照《医疗机构内新型冠状病毒感染预防与控制技术指南（第一版）》执行。

（一）医务人员进入隔离病区穿戴防护用品程序

1. 医务人员通过员工专用通道进入清洁区，认真洗手后依次戴医用防护口罩、一次性帽子或布帽、换工作鞋袜，有条件的可以更换刷手衣裤。

2. 在进入潜在污染区前穿工作服，手部皮肤有破损或疑似有损伤者戴手套进入潜在污染区。

3. 在进入污染区前，脱工作服换穿防护服或者隔离衣，加戴一次性帽子和一次性医用外科口罩（共穿戴两层帽子、口罩）、防护眼镜、手套、鞋套。

（二）医务人员离开隔离病区脱摘防护用品程序

1. 医务人员离开污染区前，应当先消毒双手，依次脱摘防护眼镜、外层一次性医用外科口罩和外层一次性帽子、防护服或者隔离衣、鞋套、手套等物品，分置于专用容器中，再次消毒手，进入潜在污染区，换穿工作服。

2. 离开潜在污染区进入清洁区前，先洗手与手消毒，脱工作服，洗手和手消毒。

3. 离开清洁区前，洗手与手消毒，摘去里层一次性帽子或布帽、里层医用防护口罩，沐浴更衣，并进行口腔、鼻腔及外耳道的清洁。

4. 每次接触患者后立即进行手的清洗和消毒。

5. 一次性医用外科口罩、医用防护口罩、防护服或者隔离衣等防护用品被患者血液、体液、分泌物等污染时应当立即更换。

6. 下班前应当进行个人卫生处置，并注意呼吸道与黏膜的防护。

（三）隔离缓冲区（医务人员更衣）的要求

医疗机构在设计隔离病房的缓冲区（医务人员更衣）时应首先考虑到医务人员穿脱个人防护用品的便捷性与舒适性，隔离缓冲区应配备手卫生设施、更衣柜、穿衣境、流程图、防护物品柜等。个人防护用品脱除区除了充分考虑污染控制的要求外，还应考虑到医务人员脱除污染防护服时身体的稳定性，如增加靠凳或靠椅。淋浴区与卫生间应设置在医务人员流程便捷处，并能保证良好的通风。

六、医用防护用品使用范围

（一）外科口罩。预检分诊、发热门诊及全院诊疗区域应当使用，需正确佩戴。污染或潮湿时随时更换。

（二）医用防护口罩。原则上在发热门诊、隔离留观病区（房）隔离病区（房）和隔离重症监护病区（房）等区域，以及进行采集呼吸道标本、气管插管、气管切开、无创通气、吸痰等可能产生气溶胶的操作时使用。一般4小时更换，污染或潮湿时随时更换。其他区城和在其他区城的诊疗操作，原则上不使用。

（三）乳胶检查手套。在预检分诊、发热门诊、隔离留观病区（房）、隔离病区（房）和隔离重症监护病区（房）等区域使用，但需正确穿戴和脱摘，注意及时更换手套。禁止戴手套离开诊疗区域戴手套不能取代手卫生。

（四）速干手消毒剂。医务人员诊疗操作过程中，手部未见明显污染物时使用，全院均应当使用。预检分诊、发热门诊、隔离留观病区（房）、隔离病区（房）和隔离重症监护病区（房）必须配备使用。

（五）护目镜。在隔离留观病区（房）、隔离病区（房）和隔离重症监护病区（房）等区域，以及采集呼吸道标本、气管插管、气管切开、无创通气、吸痰等可能出现血液、体液和分泌物等喷溅操作时使用。禁止戴着护目镜离开上述区域。如护目镜为可重复使用的，应当消毒后再复用。其他区城和在其他区城的诊疗操作原则上不使用护目镜

（六）防护面罩／防护面屏。诊疗操作中可能发生血液、体液和分泌物等

喷溅时使用。如为可重复使用的，使用后应当消毒方可再用；如为一次性使用的，不得重复使用。护目镜和防护面罩／防护面屏不需要同时使用。禁止戴着防护面罩／防护面屏离开诊疗区域。

（七）隔离衣。预检分诊、发热门诊使用普通隔离衣，隔离留观病区（房）、隔离病区（房）和隔离重症监护病区（房）使用防渗一次性隔离衣，其他科室或区域根据是否接触患者使用。一次性隔离衣不得重复使用。如使用可复用的隔离衣，使用后按规定消毒后方可再用。禁止穿着隔离衣离开上述区域。

（八）防护服。隔离留观病区（房）、隔离病区（房）和隔离重症监护病区（房）使用。防护服不得重复使用。禁止戴着医用防护口罩和穿着防护服离开上述区域。其他区域和在其他区域的诊疗操作原则上不使用防护服。

无特殊情况，符合国标（GB19082）的一次性无菌医用防护服，以及在境外上市符合日标、美标、欧标等标准的一次性无菌医用防护服（所需证明材料包括：境外医疗器械上市许可证明和检测报告、无菌证明、企业作出质量安全承诺等），仅用于隔离重症监护病区（房）等有严格微生物指标控制的场所；隔离留观病区（房）、隔离病区（房）仅使用在境外上市符合日标、美标、欧标等标准的医用防护服（所需证明材料包括：境外医疗器械上市许可证明和检测报告、企业作出质量安全承诺等），以及符合《国务院应对新型冠状病毒感染的肺炎疫情联防联控机制物资保障组关于疫情期间防护服生产使用有关问题的通知》（工信明电〔2020〕7号）中规定的"紧急医用物资防护服"。

其他人员如物业保洁人员、保安人员等需进入相关区域时，按相关区域防护要求使用防护用品，并正确穿戴和脱摘。

新冠肺炎疫情期间不同人员个人防护用品使用图表

工作岗位 ＼ 顺序	手卫生	工作帽	医用外科口罩	医用防护口罩	工作服	防护服	手套	隔离衣	防护面具/护目镜	鞋套/靴套
一般科室	●	○	●		●					
手术	●	●	●		●		●	○	○	○
预检分诊	●	●	●		●			●	○	
发热门诊	●	●	●	○	●		●	●	○	○
可能产生喷溅的操作	●	●		●	●	○	●	●	●	●
疑似/确诊患者诊疗	●	●		●		●	双层	○	●	●
疑似/确诊患者转运/陪检	●	●		●		●	●	●	●	●
疑似/确诊患者标本采集	●	●	●	●	●	●	双层	○	●	○
实验室常规检测	●	●	●		●					
实验室疑似样本检测	●	●		●	●	○	●	●		
实验室病毒核酸检测	●	●		●	●					
环境清洁消毒	●	●		●	●	●	双层 +长袖加厚橡胶手套	○	●	○
标本运送	●	●	●		●			○		
尸体处理	●	●		●	●	●	● +长袖加厚橡胶手套	○	●	●
行政管理					○					

注：1. ●应选择，○根据暴露风险选择
　　2. 暴露风险高的操作有条件时可选动力送风过滤式呼吸器

（国家卫生健康委办公厅）

附录12 新型冠状病毒肺炎防控方案（第六版）

为做好全国新型冠状病毒肺炎（以下简称新冠肺炎，COVID-19）防控工作，做到"早发现、早报告、早隔离、早治疗"，控制疫情传播，降低感染率、提高收治率，提高治愈率、降低病亡率；切实维护人民群众生命安全和身体健康，维护社会稳定，根据乙类传染病甲类管理的要求，科学防治、分区分级、精准施策，结合全国疫情形势变化及研究进展，对第五版防控方案进行修订，形成本方案。

一、目的

指导各地及时发现和报告新冠肺炎病例和聚集性疫情，开展流行病学调查和疫情处置，规范密切接触者管理，做好防控工作。

二、病原学和流行病学特征

新型冠状病毒属于 β 属冠状病毒，基因特征与 SARSR-CoV 和 MERSR-CoV 有明显区别。病毒对紫外线和热敏感，56℃ 30分钟、乙醚、75% 乙醇、含氯消毒剂、过氧乙酸和氯仿等脂溶剂均可有效灭活病毒。基于目前的流行病学调查和研究结果，潜伏期为 1 ～ 14 天，多为 3 ～ 7 天；传染源主要是新型冠状病毒感染的患者，无症状感染者也可成为传染源；主要传播途径为经呼吸道飞沫和接触传播，在相对封闭的环境中长时间暴露于高浓度气溶胶情况下存在经气溶胶传播的可能，其他传播途径尚待明确；人群普遍易感。

三、监测定义

（一）疑似病例

结合下述流行病学史和临床表现综合分析：

1. 流行病学史

（1）发病前 14 天内有武汉市及周边地区，或境内其他有病例报告的社区，或境外疫情严重国家或地区的旅行史或居住史。

（2）发病前 14 天内与新型冠状病毒感染者（核酸检测阳性者）有接触史。

（3）发病前 14 天内曾接触过来自武汉市及周边地区，或境内其他有病例报告的社区，或境外疫情严重国家或地区的发热或有呼吸道症状的患者。

（4）聚集性发病：14 天内在小范围内（如家庭、办公室、学校班级、车间等场所），出现 2 例及以上发热和 / 或呼吸道症状的病例。

2. 临床表现

（1）发热和 / 或呼吸道症状。

（2）具有新冠肺炎影像学特征。

（3）发病早期白细胞总数正常或减少，淋巴细胞计数正常或减少。

有流行病学史中的任何 1 条，且符合临床表现中任意 2 条无明确流行病学史的，符合临床表现中的 3 条。

（二）确诊病例

疑似病例，具备以下病原学或血清学证据之一者：

1. 实时荧光 RT-PCR 检测新型冠状病毒核酸阳性。

2. 病毒基因测序，与已知的新型冠状病毒高度同源。

3. 血清新型冠状病毒特异性 IgM 抗体和 IgG 抗体阳性；血清新型冠状病

毒特异性 IgG 抗体由阴性转为阳性或恢复期较急性期 4 倍及以上升高。

（三）无症状感染者

无临床症状，呼吸道等标本新型冠状病毒病原学或血清特异性 IgM 抗体检测阳性者。主要通过密切接触者筛查、聚集性疫情调查和传染源追踪调查等途径发现。

（四）聚集性疫情

聚集性疫情是指 14 天内在小范围（如家庭、办公室、学校班级、车间等）发现 2 例及以上确诊病例或无症状感染者，且存在人际传播的可能性，或共同暴露而感染的可能性。

（五）密切接触者

密切接触者指从疑似病例和确诊病例症状出现前 2 天开始，或无症状感染者标本采样前 2 天开始，未采取有效防护与其有近距离接触的人员。

四、防控措施

（一）分区分级精准防控

根据《中华人民共和国传染病防治法》《突发公共卫生事件应急条例》等法律法规，实施分区分级精准防控。以县（区）为单位，依据人口、发病情况综合研判，科学划分疫情风险等级，明确分级分类的防控策略。

1.低风险地区　实施"外防输入"策略。加强疫情严重地区以及高风险地区流入人员的跟踪管理，做好健康监测和服务。医疗机构加强发热门诊病例监测、发现、报告，疾控机构及时开展流行病学调查和密切接触者追踪管理。督促指导城乡社区、机关、企事业单位等严格落实社区防控措施，做好环境卫生整治，公众防病知识和防护技能普及等工作。

2.中风险地区　实施"外防输入、内防扩散"策略。在采取低风险地区各项措施的基础上，做好医疗救治、疾病防控相关人员、物资、场所等方面的准备，对密切接触者进行隔离医学观察和管理。以学校班级、楼房单元、工厂工作间、工作场所办公室等为最小单位，以病例发现、流行病学调查和疫情分析为线索，合理确定防控管理的场所和人员，实施针对性防控措施。无确诊病例的乡镇、街道、城乡社区可参照低风险地区采取防控措施。

3.高风险地区　实施"内防扩散、外防输出、严格管控"策略。在采取中风险地区各项措施的基础上，停止聚集性活动，依法按程序审批后可实行区域交通管控。以县域为单位，全面排查发热患者，及时收治和管理疑似病例、确诊病例和无症状感染者，对密切接触者实行隔离医学观察。对发生社区传播或聚集性疫情的城市居民小区（农村自然村）的相关场所进行消毒，采取限制人员聚集、进出等管控措施。

动态开展分析研判，及时调整风险等级，在病例数保持稳定下降、疫情扩散风险得到有效管控后，及时分地区降低应急响应级别或终止应急响应。

（二）早发现

1.各级各类医疗机构应当提高对新冠肺炎病例的诊断和报告意识，对不明原因发热、干咳等呼吸道症状或腹泻等消化道症状的病例，结合其流行病学史，及时组织院内专家会诊或主诊医师会诊，并采集标本进行病原学检测。

2.基层相关组织或用工单位对近14天内有武汉市及周边地区，或境内有病例报告的社区，或境外疫情严重国家或地区的旅行史或居住史的人员，做好健康监测；对于出现发热、干咳等呼吸道症状或腹泻等消化道症状者，作为重点风险人群进行筛查，由专业机构采样检测

3. 利用全国不明原因肺炎监测、流感样病例监测和住院严重急性呼吸道感染病例监测等现有监测网络，强化病原学监测。

4. 加强口岸卫生检疫，严格实施口岸体温监测和医学巡查，对出现发热、干咳等呼吸道症状或腹泻等消化道症状的人员加强流行病学调查和医学排查，按要求采样检测。

5. 对密切接触者做好健康监测，对于出现发热、干咳等呼吸道症状或腹泻等消化道症状者，及时转运至定点医疗机构，并采样检测。

（三）早报告

1. 病例报告　各级各类医疗卫生机构发现疑似病例、确诊病例、无症状感染者时，应当于 2 小时内进行网络直报。疾控机构在接到报告后应当立即调查核实，于 2 小时内通过网络直报系统完成报告信息的三级确认审核。不具备网络直报条件的医疗机构，应当立即向当地县（区）级疾控机构报告，并于 2 小时内将填写完成的传染病报告卡寄出；县（区）级疾控机构在接到报告后，应当立即进行网络直报，并做好后续信息的订正。

2. 报告订正　疑似病例确诊或排除后及时订正。无症状感染者如出现临床表现，及时订正为确诊病例。所有病例根据病情变化及时对临床严重程度进行订正，以病例最严重的状态为其最终状态。病例死亡后，在 24 小时内填报死亡日期。

无症状感染者的发病日期为阳性标本采集时间，诊断日期为阳性检出时间。如无症状感染者订正为确诊病例，其发病日期订正为临床症状出现的时间。

3. 突发事件的报告　根据《国家突发公共卫生事件应急预案》《国家突发公共卫生事件相关信息报告管理工作规范（试行）》要求，各县（区）出现首例新冠肺炎确诊病例、聚集性疫情，辖区疾控中心应当通过突发公共卫生事件

报告管理信息系统在 2 小时内进行网络直报，事件级别选择"未分级"。根据对事件的调查评估，及时进行调整并报告

（四）早隔离

1. 病例管理　疑似病例和确诊病例应当在定点医院隔离治疗。疑似病例单人单间隔离治疗，连续两次新型冠状病毒核酸检测阴性（采样时间至少间隔 24 小时）且发病 7 天后新型冠状病毒特异性 IgM 和 IgG 抗体仍为阴性可排除疑似病例诊断。

2. 出院后管理　病例符合出院标准，出院后建议继续进行 14 天的隔离管理和健康状况监测。鼓励有条件的省份加强出院病例随访和呼吸道标本样本检测，检测阳性者需集中隔离医学观察，并将相关信息报送中国疾控中心。

3. 无症状感染者管理　无症状感染者应集中隔离 14 天，原则上两次连续标本核酸检测阴性者（采样时间至少间隔 24 小时）可解除隔离。

（五）早治疗

各级各类医疗机构对诊断的疑似病例要及时转运至定点医院，定点医院应当做好医疗救治所需的人员、药品、设施、设备、防护用品等准备工作，按照最新版新型冠状病毒肺炎诊疗方案进行规范救治，做到应隔尽隔、应收尽收、应检尽检、应治尽治，提高收治率和治愈率，降低感染率和病亡率。

（六）流行病学调查

按照属地化管理原则，由病例就诊医疗机构所在的县（区）级卫生健康行政部门组织疾控机构开展流行病学调查，国家支持采用信息化的手段开展调查、分析和研判。

1. 个案调查　县（区）级疾控机构接到报告后，应当于 24 小时内完成病

例和无症状感染者的流行病学调查。具体要求按照中国疾控中心印发的新冠肺炎流行病学调查指南执行，并根据中国疾控中心制定的新冠肺炎病例密切接触者调查与管理指南的要求做好密切接触者的判定和登记；做好疑似病例基本信息和其密切接触者登记。

2. 聚集性疫情调查 县（区）级疾控机构根据网络直报信息和病例个案调查情况，对符合定义的聚集性疫情立即开展调查。具体要求按照中国疾控中心印发的新冠肺炎流行病学调查指南执行。

3. 信息报告 县（区）级疾控机构完成确诊病例、无症状感染者个案调查或聚集性疫情调查后，将个案调查表和调查报告及时通过网络报告系统进行上报。

（七）密切接触者追踪和管理

县（区）级卫生健康行政部门会同相关部门组织实施密切接触者的追踪和管理。对密切接触者实行集中隔离医学观察，不具备条件的地区可采取居家隔离医学观察，每日至少进行2次体温测定，并询问是否出现发热、干咳等呼吸道症状或腹泻等消化道症状。密切接触者医学观察期为与病例或无症状感染者末次接触后14天。疑似病例排除后，其密切接触者可解除医学观察。具体要求按照中国疾控中心制定的新冠肺炎病例密切接触者调查与管理指南执行。

（八）标本采集和实验室检测

收治病例的医疗机构要及时采集病例相关的临床标本。承担标本检测的机构（符合条件的医疗机构、疾控机构或第三方检测机构）应在12小时内反馈实验室检测结果。标本采集、运送、存储和检测严格按照中国疾控中心印发的新冠肺炎实验室检测技术指南要求执行。

各地区新冠肺炎 5 例及以上的聚集性病例，以及境外输入病例的所有原始标本应当送至中国疾控中心进行复核。

（九）重点场所、机构、人群防控

强化多部门联防联控工作机制，最大限度减少公众聚集性活动，因地制宜落实车站、机场、码头、商场、公共卫生间等公众场所和汽车、火车、飞机等密闭交通工具的通风、消毒、体温监测等措施。

企业复工复产后，指导企业组织员工有序返岗，做好通风、消毒、体温监测等防控工作，为员工配备必要的个人防护用品，采取分区作业、分散就餐等方式，有效减少人员聚集。指导做好农民工的健康教育和返岗复工前体温检测工作，发现异常情况，及时报告处置，加强排查识别，阻断风险人员外出。

学校、托幼机构复课复园后，指导做好返校师生的健康提示和健康管理及教室的通风、消毒等工作，督促落实入学入托晨（午）检和因病缺课（勤）病因追查与登记等防控措施。接到疫情报告后及时开展流行病学调查及疫情处置，指导做好区域消毒等工作。

指导养老机构、残障人员福利机构以及监管场所等特殊机构进一步规范出入人员管理，严格通风、日常清洁、消毒等卫生措施，加强个人防护，健康监测与管理，做好失能半失能人群日常管理等工作。

落实来华（归国）人员口岸卫生检疫，加强对疫情严重国家和地区来华（归国）人员健康管理，做好疑似病例、确诊病例、密切接触者等重点人员的排查、诊治和医学观察，严防疫情跨境传播。

（十）院内感染控制、特定场所消毒和人员防护

医疗机构应当按照医疗机构内新型冠状病毒感染预防与控制技术指南的要求，严格做好院内感染控制。同时，严格按照《医疗机构消毒技术规范》《医

院空气净化管理规范》做好医疗器械、污染物品、物体表面、地面和空气等的清洁与消毒。根据《医疗废物管理条例》《医疗卫生机构医疗废物管理办法》做好医疗废物的处置和管理。

做好病例和无症状感染者居住过的场所（如家庭、医疗机构隔离病房、转运工具以及医学观察场所等特定场所）的消毒，做好流行病学调查、隔离病区及医学观察场所工作人员和参与病例转运、尸体处理、环境清洁消毒、标本采集和实验室工作等特定人群的防护，具体要求按照中国疾控中心印发的特定场所消毒技术指南和特定人群个人防护指南执行。

（十一）宣传教育与风险沟通

普及新冠肺炎防控知识，加强重点人群健康教育，通过多种途径做好公众个人防护指导，减少人群中可能的接触或暴露。根据疫情防控进展和对新冠肺炎认识的加深，及时调整健康教育策略组织科普宣传。积极开展舆情监测，及时向公众解疑释惑，回应社会关切，做好疫情防控风险沟通工作。

五、保障措施

（一）加强组织领导

各地政府加强对本地疫情防控工作的领导，落实防控资金和物资，按照"预防为主、防治结合、科学指导、及时救治"的工作原则，全面做好新冠肺炎防控工作。

（二）强化联防联控

加强部门间信息共享，定期会商研判疫情发展趋势。各级卫生健康行政部门负责疫情控制的总体指导工作。各级疾控机构负责开展病例监测、流行病学调查和密切接触者管理及实验室检等工作。各级各类医疗机构负责病例的发现与报告、隔离、诊断、救治和临床管理，开展标本采集工作，做好院内感染防控。

（三）加强能力建设

对医疗卫生机构的专业人员开展新冠肺炎专业技术培训，强化预防为主，关口前移。加强科学研究，发挥信息技术在传染病防控中的作用，广泛开展新冠肺炎传播特点、临床特征、策略评估等相关调查，为优化防控策略提供科学证据。在传染病预防和救治工作中，鼓励、支持发挥中医中药的作用。

（国家卫生健康委办公厅）

附录 13 国家卫生健康委办公厅关于做好新型冠状病毒感染的肺炎疫情期间医疗机构医疗废物管理工作的通知

各省、自治区、直辖市及新疆生产建设兵团卫生健康委：

为做好新型冠状病毒感染的肺炎疫情期间医疗废物管理工作，有效防止疾病传播，按照《传染病防治法》《医疗废物管理条例》和《医疗卫生机构医疗废物管理办法》等法律法规规定，现将有关要求通知如下：

一、落实医疗机构主体责任

医疗机构要高度重视新型冠状病毒感染的肺炎疫情期间医疗废物管理，切实落实主体责任，其法定代表人是医疗废物管理的第一责任人，产生医疗废物的具体科室和操作人员是直接责任人。实行后勤服务社会化的医疗机构要加强对提供后勤服务机构和人员的管理，组织开展培训，督促其掌握医疗废物管理的基本要求，切实履行职责。加大环境卫生整治力度，及时处理产生的医疗废物，避免各种废弃物堆积，努力创造健康卫生环境。

二、加强医疗废物的分类收集

（一）明确分类收集范围。医疗机构在诊疗新型冠状病毒感染的肺炎患者及疑似患者发热门诊和病区（房）产生的废弃物，包括医疗废物和生活垃圾，均应当按照医疗废物进行分类收集。

（二）规范包装容器。医疗废物专用包装袋、利器盒的外表面应当有警示标识，在盛装医疗废物前，应当进行认真检查，确保其无破损、无渗漏。医废物收集桶应为脚踏式并带盖。医疗废物达到包装袋或者利器盒的3/4时，应当有效封口，确保封口严密。应当使用双层包装袋盛装医疗废物，采用鹅颈结式封口，分层封扎。

（三）做好安全收集。按照医疗废物类别及时分类收集，确保人员安全，控制感染风险。盛装医疗废物的包装袋和利器盒的外表面被感染性废物污染时，应当增加一层包装袋。分类收集使用后的一次性隔离衣、防护服等物品时，严禁挤压。每个包装袋、利器盒应当系有或粘贴中文标签，标签内容包括：医疗废物产生单位、产生部门、产生日期、类别，并在特别说明中标注"新型冠状病毒感染的肺炎"或者简写为"新冠"。

（四）分区域进行处理。收治新型冠状病毒感染的肺炎患者及疑似患者发热门诊和病区（房）的潜在污染区和污染区产生的医疗废物，在离开污染区前应当对包装袋表面采用1000mg/L的含氯消毒液喷洒消毒（注意喷洒均匀）或在其外面加套一层医疗废物包装袋；清洁区产生的医疗废物按照常规的医疗废物处置。

（五）做好病原标本处理。医疗废物中含病原体的标本和相关保存液等高危险废物，应当在产生地点进行压力蒸汽灭菌或者化学消毒处理，然后按照感染性废物收集处理。

三、加强医疗废物的运送贮存

（一）安全运送管理。在运送医疗废物前，应当检查包装袋或者利器盒的标识、标签以及封口是否符合要求。工作人员在运送医疗废物时，应当防止造成医疗废物专用包装袋和利器盒的破损，防止医疗废物直接接触身体，避免医疗废物泄漏和扩散。每天运送结束后，对运送工具进行清洁和消毒，含氯消毒液浓度为1000mg/L；运送工具被感染性医疗废物污染时，应当及时消毒处理。

（二）规范贮存交接。医疗废物暂存处应当有严密的封闭措施，设有工作人员进行管理，防止非工作人员接触医疗废物。医疗废物宜在暂存处单独设置区域存放，尽快交由医疗废物处置单位进行处置。用 1000mg/L 的含氯消毒液对医疗废物暂存处地面进行消毒，每天两次。医疗废物产生部门、运送人员、暂存处工作人员以及医疗废物处置单位转运人员之间，要逐层登记交接，并说明其来源于新型冠状病毒感染的肺炎患者或疑似患者。

（三）做好转移登记。严格执行危险废物转移联单管理，对医疗废物进行登记。登记内容包括医疗废物的来源、种类、重量或者数量、交接时间、最终去向以及经办人签名，特别注明"新型冠状病毒感染的肺炎"或"新冠"，登记资料保存 3 年。

医疗机构要及时通知医疗废物处置单位进行上门收取，并做好相应记录。各级卫生健康行政部门和医疗机构要加强与生态环境部门、医疗废物处置单位的信息互通，配合做好新型冠状病毒感染的肺炎疫情期间医疗废物的规范处置。

国家卫生健康委办公厅

2020 年 1 月 28 日

Chapter 1   Prevention and Control Management in Leishenshan Hospital

Part 1   Construction Site and Principles of Infection Prevention and Control

1.Site of Hospital

Wuhan Leishenshan Hospital is one of the infectious disease hospitals with the largest number of beds for COVID-19 patients in China, and it is also the largest temporary hospital in China. It is located in Jiangxia District, at Huangjia Lake. To the north is the military Road and to the east is Huangjiahu Avenue. The hospital was constructed as a field hospital and is designed in accordance with the standards for infectious disease hospitals, with modular and standardized installation and construction. The hospital covers an area of 21.9 hectares, with a total building area of 79,900 square meters, which has 1,500 beds and accommodates about 2,300 medical staff.

2.Design of Prevention and Control Management

2.1 Overall Design Concept of Prevention and Control Management

In theory, the external environment of the hospital includes a separation with a distance of at least 20 meters between the isolation zone and the surrounding roads and buildings, as per the requirements of infectious disease hospitals. Principally, nosocomial infection prevention and control management require a clear division between living quarters and wards, clear logistics and traffic lines, and shunting for contaminants and cleansers (Table 1.1). The hospital area includes three major functional areas: medical isolation area, medical living area and logistics support area (Figure 1.1).

The isolation area is divided into north and south area. The north area (Area A) contains 15 wards, 1 ICU, an operating field, and 2 medical technology areas. The south area contains 3 wards and 1 ICU in Area B and 12 wards in Area C. All wards are equipped with oxygen supply system and negative pressure suction system, which meet various functions of the infectious disease hospital. The design layout of the medical isolation area is "fishbone-like". The "main bone" is the main road for medical care in the wards. This road enters and exits the medical care entrance and is provided with a sanitary passage. "Branches" are the isolation wards, each of which is built as standardized ward units. These wards contain: the first dressing room, the second dressing room, personal protective equipment (PPE) room, treatment room, nursing station, pharmacy, doctor's office, clean aisle, buffer zone, isolation aisle, standardized ward, outer aisle, instrument room, medical waste temporary storage, reception room, disposal room, specimen room, pantry, etc.

The medical living area includes office building, medical living building, cleaning supplies warehouse and logistics area. A 20 meters isolation green belt separates the living area and the isolation area.

The logistics support area is equipped with sewage treatment, medical waste incineration, medical waste temporary storage, positive and negative pressure station buildings, liquid oxygen station, rainwater collection pond, and ambulance disinfection station, etc.

Table 1.1   Factors to graphic design of hospital

Sort	Factor
Environment	Clear shunting for contaminants and cleansers, doctors and patients, pedestrian flow and traffic stream

Continuous the table

Sort	Factor
Building	Lighting, sanitation, ventilation, sunshine, fire prevention
Protection	Medical waste disposal area
Control	4 entrances to the hospital
	Ambulance decontamination at the patient's main entrance

2.2 Design of the Negative Pressure Isolation Unit

For the safety of doctors and patients, negative pressure systems are installed in the isolation wards, medical technology departments and operating rooms. All wards are sealed and natural ventilation is not allowed since the airflow should be accurately controlled. Negative pressure isolation ward requires ventilation for at least 12 times per hour, and the pressure difference between the ward and the buffer room is kept about −5Pa to −10Pa, creating an increasing gradient pressure in the order of the ward toilet, ward, buffer room, inner corridor, buffer room, and office. This pressure gradient makes the air flow from the clean area to the potentially polluted area and finally to the polluted area. It also prevents backflow of air. The ward, the buffer room and the inner corridor are equipped with pressure gauges to monitor pressure at any time.

The air supply system contains with three–stage filters of rough, medium and sub–high efficiency to ensure clean air along the ceiling. Also, the exhaust system is equipped with three levels of rough, medium and high–efficiency filters to block dust and pathogens from the ward. This ensures the exhaust air meets the requirements of biological safety and environmental protection. The exhaust port is installed at the patient's bedside, and the low edge of which is below 0.1m to the ground and the high edge does not go beyond 0.6m to the ground.

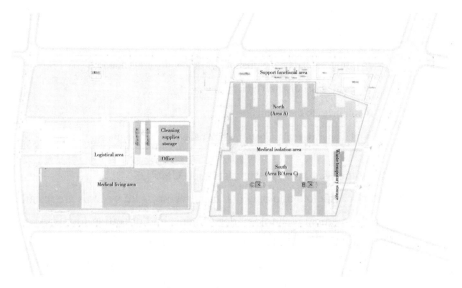

Figure 1.1　General plan of Leishenshan Hospital

Part 2　Layout of Leishenshan Hospital

1. Planning Layout

Overall, the architectural layout of the Leishenshan Hospital fully complies with the design of infectious disease hospitals "three zones and two passages". It is strictly divided into clean passages and contaminated passages. Patients and medical staff entrances are strictly separated. Also, contaminants and cleansers entrances are sternly distinguished. The clean channels are mainly used by medical staff, as the passage for cleaning and maintenance personnel, transport of cleaning supplies, the disinfected quilt, and the sterilized items, etc. Contaminated channels are mainly used by patients, medical waste transfer and specimen transfer, etc. Clean and contaminated channels are prohibited from retrograde motion. People entering a polluted channel from a clean channel must wear PPE and follow the designated route. Similarly, people working in the polluted area entering potentially polluted area or clean aisle, must remove PPE and undergo sanitation (Figure 1.2).

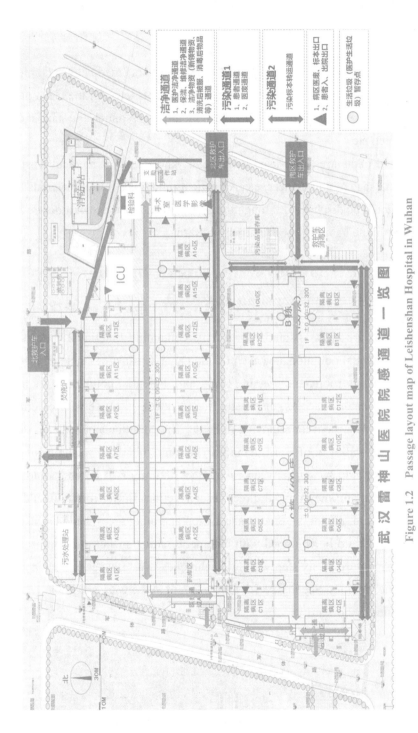

Figure 1.2   Passage layout map of Leishenshan Hospital in Wuhan

2. Movement Path in Hospital

The clean paths include those used by all workers (medical staffs, cleaners, repairing works, ect.) and to transport sanitary materials, etc. All the clean passages in the hospital are limited to military road–medical personnel entrance and exit–medical street, etc.

Polluted paths are those used by patients, and transport medical wastes and specimen, passage of ambulances, etc. All patients and other waster materials leaving the ward should be discharged through the patient's entrance and exit doors, and the same route should be used when returning to ward.

Part 3　Layout of the Process of Infection Prevention and Control in Leishenshan Hospital

All wards are built as standardized units containing functional zones such as clean area, potential pollution area and pollution area. Clean areas include: rest room, duty room, bathing room, and dressing PPE room. Potential pollution areas include: nurse station, material access, dispensing room, doctor's office with external and internal aisle, and a room for removing PPE, etc. The pollution area include: isolation ward, external walkway of ward, temporary storage of waste, washing room, etc. Buffer room should be set between each zone, and any two doors should not be opened at the same time to avoid direct air convection. Buffer rooms should be set outside each ward, doctor's office, nurse station and other areas, hand basins. These buffer rooms should be equipped with automatic induction faucets, hand sanitizer, hand towels, picture of six step washing techniques, waste paper baskets and other hand hygiene facilities. See Figure 1.3 for the layout of the ward and Table 1.2 for the main activities in the ward.

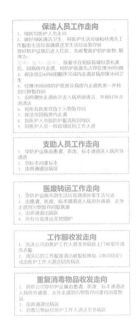
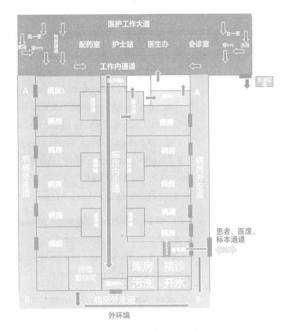

Figure 1.3   Passage layout of Leishenshan Hospital ward

Table 1.2   The main activities in Leishenshan Hospital (Combined with Figure 1.3)

Work	The process
Medical staff	1.The medical staff must go to work through the cleanly path 2.When the medical staff leave ward, they should wear PPE and go through the patient access
Cleaner	1. They should abide by the medical staff route when working 2. Keep the clean and potential pollution areas clean 3. After wearing the protective equipment, they should enter the deprotection buffer room in reverse order, first collect the medical protection waste, in the order of; buffer room 3, buffer room 2, buffer room 1, and pack it in the corresponding area as per the requirements, then return to the internal walkway of the ward, and put the protective medical waste into side B of the buffer room 4. The cleaner completes the sanitation of the internal walkway and the buffer room of the ward in the order of A to B

Continuous the table

Work	The process
	5. Transfer the protective medical waste and corridor waste in the ward to the waste temporary storage place through buffer room B 6. Enter the ward from the external walkways to clean the external walkways 7. Store all medical waste in the waste storage room 8. The cleaner goes back to the internal corridor in the ward 9. Return to green area after taking off protective clothing according to the process of medical staff 10. Goes back to the Work Avenue from green area following medical staff
Support staff	1. Enter the external walkways passage of the ward from the clean area after wearing protective equipment 2. Collect specimen and put them in the specimen room 3. Return from the original way
Clinic waste transportation	1. Collect domestic waste from the domestic waste aisle after wearing protective equipment 2. Enter temporary storage room to collect clinic waste from the external walkways passage of the ward though the patients' aisles, medical waste aisle or specimens aisles 3. Return from the original road 4. Put all solid wastes to incinerator
Receiving and dispatching work clothes	1. Workers from a washing company arrives in each ward to collect the laundry from the medical avenue 2. The clean working clothes should be placed in the clothing station (location to be determined) or sent back to each ward through the medical avenue
Reusable sterilized materials	1. Workers from the disinfection company collect the items to be disinfected which are placed in temporary storage room from the external walkways of the ward through the patients aisles, medical waste aisle or specimens aisles after wearing protective equipment 2. The workers return through the original road 3. The sterilized materials are sent to each ward from the medical avenue

(Fu Qiao　Ying Wang　Di Shi　Xiao-ping Zhu)

Chapter 2　The Organization Structure of Nosocomial Infection Management in Leishenshan Hospital

Part 1　Organization Structure

Establish a complete system of the management organization structure of nosocomial infection, and set up a Nosocomial Infection Management Committee. The committee constitutes the director serving as the chairperson, the deputy director in charge of medical service as the vice–chairperson, each medical team leader as the main member, and the invited members of the National Health Commission Wuhan Nosocomial Infection Management Expert Group as consultants. The Nosocomial Infection Management Committee has an executive committee comprising of the chairperson who is the deputy director in charge of the medical treatment, the nosocomial infection management team, and the heads of nosocomial infection management in each ward as members (Figure 2.1). Wuhan Leishenshan Hospital implements a Large Department System; the medical management department is composed of the nosocomial infection management team, medical teams, nursing teams, comprehensive coordination groups, and other departments responsible for the medical service work. Based on the actual conditions in each ward, their respective medical teams have set up a nosocomial infection prevention and control team consisting of the head of the department, participation of the head nurse, and the infection control professionals (Figure 2.2).

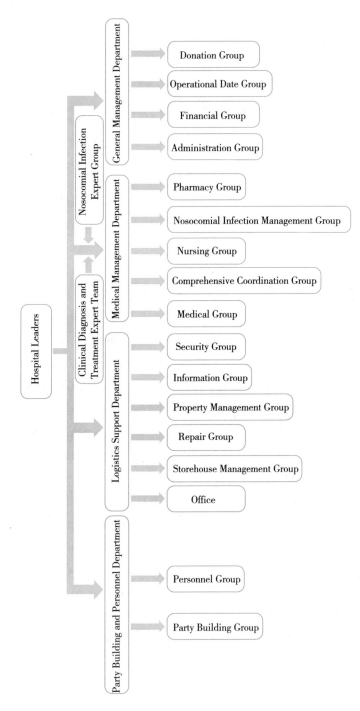

Figure 2.1   The administrative structure of Leishenshan Hospital

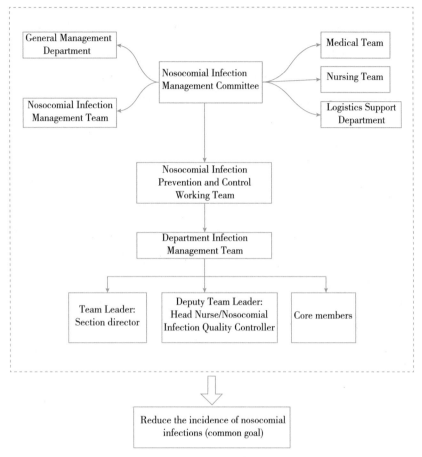

Figure 2.2   The three−level architecture diagram of nosocomial infection
management of the Leishenshan Hospital

Part 2   Duties of the Nosocomial Infection Management Committee

1. The Nosocomial Infection Management Committee formulates plans, standards, systems, monitoring measures, and specific implementation measures for the prevention and control of nosocomial infection as per the national laws and regulations.

2. During the prevention and control of COVID-19, the Nosocomial Infection Management Committee supervises, inspects, directs, and consults on the management of nosocomial infection.

3. Research and decide on major decisions and critical matters related to emergency work on nosocomial infection in the prevention and control of COVID-19, direct and dispatch various hospital resources to be involved in medical treatment, and decide to start, change, or terminate the hospital emergency response level.

4. The Nosocomial Infection Management Committee regularly holds working meetings to summarize work, analyze problems, arrange tasks, and promptly provide opinions, and suggestions to the hospital leaders and relevant departments on the existing issues, for the effective implementation of the nosocomial infection prevention and control measures.

5. Responsible for coordinating the nosocomial infection prevention and control work in all departments of the hospital, and provide business technical guidance.

6. Execute other crucial matters related to nosocomial infection prevention and control.

Part 3　Composition and Duties of the Nosocomial Infection Management Team

1.Composition

The staffing of the Office of the Nosocomial Infections Prevention and Control Management of the newly built infectious disease hospital is reasonably allocated as per the number of beds. The Wuhan Leishenshan Hospital plans 1500 beds and assigns 6 nosocomial infection prevention and control personnel at 250 beds per person. While building and receiving the current situation of patients, the nosocomial infection management team was urgently recruited from the clinical department, and other departments in the initial stage of the establishment and currently, there 13 full-time nosocomial infection staff. Based on this, a reserve 40 part-time staff for nosocomial infection prevention and control were trained. These 40 nosocomial infection prevention and control part-time staffs have undergone a month-long intensive training in theory and practice, and are primarily responsible for the nosocomial infection prevention and serve as the control supervisors in each ward.

2.Work Responsibilities

2.1 Under the leader of the Nosocomial Infection Management Committee, responsible for the daily work of nosocomial infection management.

2.2 The nosocomial infection management team reviews and provides guidelines in the architectural layout, basic layout of the critical departments, basic facilities, and work procedures of the hospital as per the nosocomial infection prevention and control and hygienic requirements for COVID-19 of the National and Provincial Health committees.

2.3 Research and determine the key departments, key links, key processes, risk factors, and intervention measures for nosocomial infection prevention and control in hospitals, and clarify the responsibilities of the relevant departments and personnel in the prevention and control of nosocomial infection.

2.4 Responsible for formulation and promulgation of relevant rules and regulations for the prevention and control of nosocomial infection of COVID-19, as well as supervising and inspecting their implementation.

2.5 Responsible for the promotion of nosocomial infection prevention and control of COVID-19, and train all medical teams on nosocomial infection prevention and control.

2.6 Responsible for the prevention and control plan of nosocomial infection prevention and control of COVID-19, and organize its implementation.

2.7 Regularly report to the Nosocomial Infection Management Committee to study, discuss, and analyze the current status of nosocomial infection prevention and control, to target infection factors, including the current state of infection control, deploy work, and formulate measures. In exceptional circumstances, the team shall call for a meeting at any given time.

2.8 Regularly monitor the environment of each department in the hospital, management of sterile materials, operation of aseptic technology, hand hygiene, disinfection and isolation protection, management of reused medical devices, disposal of medical waste, put forward rectification opinions, and urge the implementation of rectification.

2.9 Responsible for the registration, guidance, verification, and protection of the occupational exposure of the medical personnel.

Part 4   Composition and Duties of the Nosocomial Infection Management Team of the Clinical Department

1. Based on the requirements of the nosocomial infection control team, a clinical department nosocomial infection management team with clear responsibilities is set up to be responsible for the nosocomial infection management work of the undergraduate department. The team personnel have clear responsibilities and implement them.

2. Staffing

2.1 The person in charge of the clinical department is the first person responsible for nosocomial infection management in the ward.

2.2 The members of the nosocomial infection management team of the clinical department include physicians and nurses. There is a full-time staff member of the nosocomial infection management who is a permanent staff in the ward.

3. Duties

3.1 The infection prevention and quality control team in the clinical department is responsible for the various tasks of nosocomial infection management of the undergraduate department. Based on the characteristics of the infection prevention and control in the hospital of the undergraduate department, the corresponding nosocomial infection management system is formulated and implemented.

3.2 Cooperate with the infection management department of the hospital to monitor and control COVID–19, and other infectious diseases in this ward, and regularly conduct self–examination and analysis on the prevention and control of COVID–19. Identify problems and improve in time.

3.3 Responsible for the training of the permanent and temporary staff of the department in nosocomial infection management knowledge and skills.

3.4 Accept the supervision, inspection, and guidance of the nosocomial infection management work of the department, implement the relevant improvement measures of nosocomial infection management, evaluate the improvement effect, and make corresponding records of the hospital.

4. Duties of Nosocomial Infection Quality Controller

4.1 The quality controller is appointed by the director of the department and the head nurse in this department as a fixed and responsible person. It is recommended that the department organizes for full–time work in nosocomial infection prevention and control in the department.

4.2 Responsible for the implementation of all nosocomial infection management tasks in the department under the guidance of the nosocomial infection management team, section director, and the head nurse.

4.3 Communicate nosocomial infection prevention, and control systems, procedures and notifications promptly. Participate in the formulation of various nosocomial infection management systems and be responsible for the implementation.

4.4 Supervise and guide the implementation of various nosocomial infection management systems. Guide the configuration of various disinfectant solutions and monitor the concentration of disinfectant solutions and quality.

4.5 Responsible for supervising and guiding the dressing of medical, consultation, and logistics staff, etc.

4.6 Responsible for the timely collection and replenishment of various medical protective articles, disinfection drugs, and related articles in the department.

4.7 Responsible for training on nosocomial infection prevention and control knowledge, occupational hazards, and protective measures. Responsible for the training of newly admitted staff on nosocomial infection prevention and control knowledge and training records.

4.8 Responsible for training and recording of cleaning, disinfection, and isolation knowledge for sanitation workers, checking and guiding the implementation of cleaning and sanitation work by sanitation workers.

4.9 Provide timely feedback to the section director and head nurse regarding issues in the prevention and control of nosocomial infections in the department.

4.10 Attend meetings and training organized by the nosocomial infection management team and submit relevant reports on time.

5. Staff Responsibilities

5.1 Actively participate in the training on knowledge and skills related to nosocomial infection management.

5.2 Follow and implement all protection standards, procedures, and requirements issued by the nosocomial infection management committee.

5.3 Conduct surveillance of nosocomial infection of COVID–19 and report according to the requirements of the hospital.

5.4 Learn about the prevention and control of nosocomial infection of COVID–19.

5.5 Follow the aseptic technique operation procedures when engaged in aseptic technique diagnosis and treatment operations, including injection, treatment, and drug changing, etc.

5.6 Follow the national management principles for the rational use of antibacterials and use them reasonably. Supervise and guide cleaning staff and security staff to acquire the knowledge and skills about cleaning, disinfection, and protection related to their job.

(Xiao–ping Zhu   Yi–ping Mao   Lu Gan   Di Shi)

Chapter 3　Nosocomial Infection Prevention, Control Regulations and Standard Operating Procedures

Part 1　Nosocomial Infection Prevention, Control Regulations and Contingency Plan

1. Nosocomial Infection Prevention and Control System in the Isolation Wards

1.1 Establish nosocomial infection management team in the wards, which is responsible for nosocomial infection management. Group members should have clear responsibilities and implement all the nosocomial infection prevention and control protocols.

1.1.1 Management requirements

A nosocomial infection management team with clear responsibilities should be established to take charge of nosocomial infection management in the ward. The members of the team should have clear responsibilities and implement them accordingly.

1.1.2 Personnel form

ⅰ. The person in charge of the ward is the key person responsible for nosocomial infection management.

ⅱ. The nosocomial infection management team includes doctors and nurses.

ⅲ. The members of the nosocomial infection management team should be relatively fixed, and the doctors should have credentials of the attending physician or above.

1.1.3 Responsibilities

ⅰ. The nosocomial infection management team is responsible for all aspects of infection prevention, control and management in the ward. Based on the nature of the nosocomial infection, the prevention and control team in the ward should develop corresponding nosocomial infection prevention and control management systems and establish implementation.

ⅱ. The nosocomial infection management team should cooperate with the infection control and quality control department of the hospital to carry out nosocomial infection prevention and control monitoring in the ward. The nosocomial infection cases should be reported in a timely manner, and regular self-examination and analysis conducted to implement medical infection monitoring, prevention and control to identify problems and improve them in time. Corresponding records should be made.

ⅲ. The team is responsible for training information and skills on nosocomial infection management of staff in the ward.

ⅳ. The team should accept hospital supervision, inspection and guidance on nosocomial infection management in the ward, implement the relevant improvement nosocomial infection management measures, evaluate the improvement effect and make corresponding records.

1.1.4 Staff members

ⅰ. Actively participate in training on knowledge and skills related to nosocomial infection management.

ⅱ. Observe the standard prevention principles and implement specific measures for standard prevention. Hand hygiene should be done according to requirements of WS/T313; isolation should follow the requirements of WS/T311; disinfection and sterilization should follow the requirements of WS/T367.

ⅲ. Follow the hospital and the ward related protocols for prevention and control of infection.

ⅳ. Carry out surveillance of nosocomial infection prevention and control and report according to the hospital requirements.

ⅴ. When engaged in aseptic diagnosis and treatment operations, such as injection, treatment, and dressing changing, etc., aseptic technique operation procedures should be followed.

ⅵ. The cleaners, catering staff, etc. should have knowledge and skills on their work related cleaning and disinfection.

1.1.5 Education and training

ⅰ. The ward nosocomial infection management team should regularly organize training on nosocomial infection management and make assessment for the medical staff in the ward.

ⅱ. The ward nosocomial infection management team should regularly evaluate the cleaning staffs' knowledge on nosocomial infection prevention and control such as cleaning and disinfection, hand hygiene, personal protection, etc., as well as carry out corresponding training and guidance according to their knowledge.

ⅲ. The ward nosocomial infection management team should publicize and educate patients, escorts, and other relevant personnel on nosocomial infection prevention and control related information such as hand hygiene and isolation.

1.2 Work requirements

The prevention and control of nosocomial infection in quarantine wards should be carried out in accordance with the nosocomial infection prevention and control system, the ward disinfection system, the ward medical staff protection system, and the ward monitoring system.

1.2.1 The layout of the ward should be realistic, the zoning clear, the environment kept tidy, regularly cleaned and disinfected.

1.2.2 Staff from outside the ward are not allowed. If they must enter, they should get permission from the medical staff in the ward and accept the isolation protection requirement guidance, strictly abide to the related requirements of isolation protection, and make clear registration records.

1.2.3 When medical personnel enters the ward, they should be properly protected according to the requirements of the work area. Their clothes and hats should be kept clean, and aseptic technical procedures and hand hygiene related systems should be strictly implemented during their operation.

1.2.4 Medical personnel should wear appropriate personal protective equipment (gloves, masks, caps, etc.), and each patient should wash his hands or disinfect them. Personal protective equipment should be changed every shift, and replaced in case of contamination.

1.2.5 Strictly implement hand hygiene related systems and requirements, wash hands properly and improve hand hygiene management.

1.2.6 It is strictly forbidden to wear protective equipment in the hospital outside the ward. When going out, one should take off work clothes or protective equipment, wear personal clothes or clothes for going out when leaving the ward.

1.2.7 Visitors are not allowed in the wards.

2. Nosocomial Infection Surveillance System

Hospitals must carry out infection monitoring on patients in order to grasp the incidence of nosocomial infection, multiple locations, multiple departments, high-risk factors, pathogen characteristics, and drug resistance, etc., so as to provide scientific basis for nosocomial infection control.

2.1 Hospitals should adopt a proactive monitoring method for comprehensive monitoring.

2.1.1 The nosocomial infection management team must summarize and analyze the monitoring data on a monthly basis, report regularly to the Nosocomial Infection Management Committee. The Nosocomial Infection Management Working Committee should report back to the hospital's medical staff. The monitoring data should be properly stored, and special instances should be reported in time.

2.1.2 Early warning and surveillance of outbreak nosocomial infection should be implemented. Problems should be identified in time and reported directly to the in charge.

2.1.3 Hospitals should monitor diseases other than the novel coronavirus and timely report any infectious diseases according to the requirements of infectious disease management.

2.1.4 Hospitals should gradually carry out surveillance through nosocomial infection information, and regularly analyze the trend of surveillance data.

2.2 Hospitals should carry out targeted surveillance on the basis of comprehensive surveillance. The surveillance goals should be determined by the characteristics of the hospital, the priorities and difficulties of the nosocomial infection control.

2.3 The target monitoring data should be analyzed and regular feedback provided. Its effect should be evaluated, and improved measures should be proposed; there should be periodic summary reports; complete the monitoring should and a final report.

2.4 Hospitals must regularly monitor the effectiveness of disinfection. The sterilization pass rate must reach 100%, and unqualified items should be exempted from the clinical department.

2.5 Environmental Hygiene Monitoring: monitoring of air, surface of objects, and hands of medical staff should be implemented.

2.6 Each ward should strictly carry out various surveillance in accordance to the requirements of *Infection Surveillance Contents of Hospital of Wuhan Leishenshan Hospital* (Appendix 1 for details).

3. Full-time Work System of Nosocomial Infection Prevention and Control Monitoring in the Quarantine Ward

3.1 Under the recommendation of nosocomial infection management team and the guidance of head nurse, the implementation of the nosocomial infection control system, disinfection and isolation system, and aseptic operation routine and so on should be supervised. The daily work to a specific project and the time when the project is to be completed must be refined and recorded.

3.2 For suspected or confirmed nosocomial infection, the supervising physician should report it through the intranet system of "Infection management software" in time. He/she should try to retain the corresponding specimen and send it to bacterial examination and drug sensitivity test. If 3 or more infections with the same or similar clinical symptoms occur within a short period of time during diagnosis and treatment, in case of possible epidemiologically significant co-exposure factors or co-infection sources between cases, the cases should be reported to the head of the nosocomial infection management team regardless of test results. Moreover, the head must immediately report it to the nosocomial infection management team and medical affairs officers. They help in accomplishing the epidemiological investigation and actively take control measures.

3.3 Supervise and inspect the implementation of daily disinfection, terminal disinfection, isolation and disinfection of infected patients in the isolation ward as well as protective isolation for high-risk and vulnerable populations.

3.4 Take charge of inspecting aseptic operations, quality of disinfection and isolation. Implement hand hygiene, supervise and inspect configuration and use of disinfectants as well as disinfection tools.

3.5 Monitor and record the quality of the air, object surface and medical staff hand hygiene conditions in each department according to the requirements of nosocomial infection management team.

3.6 Clean the UV lamp at least once a week.

3.7 Monitor and record disinfectant concentration in use. Timely, replace disinfectants that do not meet the standards.

3.8 Guide and supervise the daily cleaning, disinfection and medical waste transfer registration by the ward cleaners.

3.9 Implement monthly quality control according to the nosocomial infection management quality indicators.

3.10 Be in charge of nosocomial infection prevention, regulate knowledge promotion, and organize personnel in the department to participate in relevant nosocomial infection prevention and training.

3.11 Summarize, analyze and report nosocomial infection surveillance and supervision results at least once in a month, and continually improve archiving for future reference.

4. Isolation Ward Daily Cleaning and Disinfection System

4.1 Routine cleaning and disinfection specifications

4.1.1 Medical staff should remain neat and tidy during working hours. They should strictly adhere to aseptic technical operating procedures, strictly implement hand hygiene, not wear work clothes in restaurants, dormitories or outside the hospital.

4.1.2 Medical staff should use disinfectants, disinfection instruments, disposable sterile medical supplies properly. All disposable sterile medical supplies should be treated as medical waste after use.

4.1.3 Devices and supplies that come in contact with the skin and mucous membranes must be disinfected after use; medical supplies that enter human tissues or sterile organs must be sterilized.

4.1.4 Extracted sterile liquids should not be left for more than 2 hours. Opened sterile solution must be used within 2 hours. Several solvents must not exceed 24 hours after opening and the opening time should be recorded.

4.1.5 Iodine and alcohol once opened should be closed immediately after use and changed weekly. Paper-packed sterile items (cotton swab, cotton ball and gauze) should not be left for more than 4 hours once opened. The sharps box cannot be opened for more than 48 hours.

4.1.6 Cleaning tools (rag, towel) need to be clearly marked, separately washed, placed in a specific location and regularly disinfected. Do not cross-use.

4.1.7 The ward should be wet cleaned and the nightstand be wet wiped. Each towel should be used only once, soaked and infected after use. The patient bed unit should be terminally disinfected after the patient is discharged, transferred to the hospital, or dead.

4.2 Specific implementation method

4.2.1 The ward nurses and cleaning staff are jointly responsible for the daily cleaning and disinfection of the ward. The nursing team should have daily disinfection jobs, supervise personal protection of the cleaners as well as assist cleaning staff to complete cleaning and disinfection work. The head nurse of the ward is responsible for supervising these implementations.

4.2.2 Choose disposable diagnostic supplies, non-disposable diagnostic supplies should first choose pressure steam sterilization, non-heat resistant items can choose chemical disinfectants or low-temperature sterilization equipment for disinfection or disinfection.

4.2.3 Configure chlorine disinfectant as follows:

ⅰ. Chlorine disinfectant effervescent tablet (500 mg/pill): Formulated into 1000mg/L effective chlorine disinfectant.

ⅱ. Configuration method: For 500 mg/1L water, add 2 tablets and into 6 L of water, add 12 tablets.

ⅲ. After preparing the disinfectant, the effective concentration of the disinfectant concentration test chart should be used to monitor and record the effective concentration before use. Note: The chlorine-containing disinfectant once prepared should be used immediately in less than 24 hours.

4.2.4 Object surface and the ground need to be disinfected twice a day and any other time in event of contamination.

4.2.5 Disinfection method

ⅰ. Indoor air disinfection is performed using UV lamps. When using UV rays, the irradiation time should be extended to more than 1 hour.

ⅱ. The principle of cleaning before disinfection should be followed and wet sanitary cleaning method adopted.

ⅲ. Cleaning the ward, diagnosis or treatment area should be carried out in an orderly manner, from top to bottom, from the inside to the outside, from light to heavy pollution. Cleaning of wards with multiple patients should follow clean unit operations.

ⅳ. Disinfection on surface of the object should be wiped with a high-level disinfection wipe; The ground should be disinfected with 1000 mg/L effective chlorine or a 500 mg/L hydrogen peroxide disinfectant. The disinfection time should not be less than 30 minutes.

Ⅴ. When the patient's body fluid, blood or any other spillage contamination occurs during diagnosis and treatment, the stain should be cleaned and the surface disinfected immediately.

ⅵ. The specimen storage box in the ward should be wiped with 1000mg/L chlorine–containing disinfectant on the inner and outer surfaces once daily.

ⅶ. Medical waste should be handled in accordance with the requirements of *Medical waste management regulations* and *Medical and health institutions Medical waste management measures*. The use of double–layered yellow garbage bags for storage in the medical waste temporary storage room should be standardized. The staff of centralized medical waste disposal should set another layer of yellow garbage bags when transporting medical waste to the medical waste incineration station.

ⅷ. Disposal of cleaning tools after use: Rags and mops: They should be soaked and sterilized for 30 minutes in 1000 mg/L chlorine disinfectant, cleaned and dried before use. Cleaning trolley: After use, they should be pushed back to the disposal room, the body wiped with 1000 mg/L chlorine disinfectant, and then wiped with water to remove residual disinfectant before later use.

5. Terminal Disinfection System of the Isolation Ward

5.1 Timing of disinfection: Terminal disinfection refers to thorough disinfection after a source of infection leaves the relevant place. It includes disinfection of the air, the object surface and the floor of the ward after the patient is discharged, transferred to another department, or has died. The terminal disinfected site and its various items should be confirmed pathogen free. Terminal disinfection objects include pollutants (blood, secretions, vomitus, feces, etc.) discharged by patients, all appliances (including medical and nursing supplies) and the environment that may be contaminated. It is not essential to carry out large–scale outdoor environment (including air) area disinfection.

5.2 Disinfection process: routine cleaning and disinfection, as well as UV disinfection depending on the situation.

5.3 Executive staff: the on-duty medical staff in the working area is responsible for the terminal disinfection of the area, and the specific executive staff should be assigned by the department.

5.4 Disinfection method

5.4.1 Air: 0.2% peroxyacetic acid, 500 mg/L chlorine dioxide, and 3% hydrogen peroxide disinfectant can be selected independently. Ultra-low capacity spray disinfection should be carried out at 10~20 ml/m^3 dosage in 1 hour.

5.4.2 Floor and wall: Where there are visible pollutants, the pollutants should be fully removed before disinfection. When the dirt is invisible to the naked eye, it should be wiped or sprayed with 1000 mg/L chlorine disinfectant. The disinfection time should be more than 30 minutes.

5.4.3 Object surface

ⅰ.When there are visible objects on the surface of general objects, they should be cleaned before disinfection.

ⅱ.Personal electronic products can be wiped and disinfected with 75% alcohol or double-chain quaternary amine salt-containing toilet paper towels.

ⅲ.Bed frames, bedside tables, furniture, pagers, toys, bed shakers, door handles, faucets, sinks, toilet buttons, cushions, and inner and outer surfaces should be disinfected with chlorine-containing disinfectant containing 1000 mg/L effective chlorine or 500 mg/L chlorine dioxide disinfectant wipes or spray disinfectants. For multi-component combined items, such as the nightstand, the drawer and cupboard door should be opened, and both internal and external surfaces sprayed or wiped. After 30 minutes, they should be wiped clean with water.

ⅳ.Ventilator, ECMO, CT machine, monitor and other valuable equipment should be handled according to their respective procedures or instructions. Other diagnostic equipment, such as thermometers, stethoscopes, infusion pumps, blood pressure meters, oximeters, defibrillators, and other equipment surfaces based on their corrosive resistance, either 75% alcohol, 1000 mg/L chlorine-containing disinfectant or 500 mg/L chlorine dioxide can be used to wipe, soak, spray and disinfect them. After 30 minutes they should be wiped clean with water.

5.4.4 Contaminants (patient blood, secretions, vomit, and excreta): A small number of pollutants can be carefully removed by disposable absorbent materials (such as gauze, rags, etc.) with chlorine-containing disinfectant (or disinfectant wipes/dry wipes that can achieve high levels of disinfection) at 5000~10000 mg/L. A large number of pollutants should be completely covered with disinfectant powder or bleach powder containing water-absorbing ingredients, or fully covered with disposable water-absorbing materials, and then poured on a water-absorbing material with a sufficient amount of 5000 ~ 10,000mg/L chlorine-containing disinfectant for more than 30 minutes (or high level disinfection can be achieved in the towel) and carefully removed. Contact with pollutants during the cleaning process should be avoided, and the cleaned pollutants should be centrally disposed of as medical waste.

5.4.5 Disposal of fabrics: The sheets, quilts and other fabrics used by patients should be sealed in double-layer medical waste bags and incinerated as infectious medical waste. Conditioned wards can be sterilized using bed unit sterilizer.

5.4.6 Medical supplies: Use disposable diagnostic equipment, appliances and articles as much as possible. After use, they should be pre-processed, sealed in double-layer medical waste bags, and disposed of as infectious medical waste. Recyclable diagnosis and treatment equipment should be packed in double-layer medical waste bags, labeled, and put in the finishing box for disposal by the disinfection and supply center.

5.4.7 Medical waste: Handling should comply with the requirements of the Medical Waste Management Regulations and the Medical Waste Management Measures of Medical and Health Institutions, and double-layer yellow medical bag used to collect waste. When the medical waste reaches 3/4 of the package, it should be tightly sealed, sprayed and disinfected in the temporary storage room of the pollutants in the isolation area, or put into another yellow medical waste bag for transport to the incineration station.

5.4.8 Patient's items: It is recommended that items which patients do not need to take away can be incinerated as medical waste. When other personal items with no visible pollutants need to be taken away and need to be reused, they can be soaked with 500 mg/L chlorine disinfectant for 30 minutes, and then washed as usual. Other personal belongings can be irradiated by ultraviolet rays for 1 hour. Moisture-resistant items can be soaked and disinfected with 1000 mg/L disinfectant for 30 minutes. The patient's clothing, both inside and outside can be irradiated by ultraviolet rays for more than 1 hour, sealed and then stored for 14 weeks before use.

5.4.9 Corpse disposal: After the death of a patient, the movement and handling of the corpse should be minimized and it should be handled promptly by trained staff under strict protection. Chlorine-containing disinfectant (3000 ~ 5000 mg/L) cotton ball or gauze should be used to fill all open channels or wounds of the patient including mouth, nose, ears, anus, tracheotomy wound, etc. The body should be wrapped with a double-layer cloth impregnated with disinfectant and put into a double-layer body bag. The department of civil affairs should be contacted to send a special vehicle to transport the corpse for cremation as soon as possible.

6. Medical Waste Management System of COVID-19

6.1 Medical waste are mainly generated from the COVID-19 patients' and all contaminated areas, such as the isolated ward, treatment rooms, and inspection departments.

6.2 It is divided into infectious medical waste, pathological medical waste, chemical medical waste, pharmaceutical medical waste and injury medical waste.

6.3 General waste is packed in the yellow garbage bag (3/4); sharps are packed in the sharp box (3/4).

6.4 The yellow garbage bags are sealed and packed in double-layer: goose-neck layered bandages with cable ties for sealing and labeling: including source hospitals and departments, date, category (labeled as COVID-19), weight, and the number of bags.

6.5 Handover and signature: The ward personnel should weigh the waste with the transfer staff, add the third layer of the yellow medical waste bag or spray with disinfectant (1000mg / L), and then hand over and double-sign for retention.

6.6 Transport (transfer according to the designated route): The waste should be transported to the medical waste temporary storage and make a record of the transfer. Care must be taken to avoid mixing with household waste.

6.7 Incineration is carried uniformly by the hospital incinerator.

7. Occupational Exposure Management System

7.1 Protective measures for medical staff to prevent COVID-19 infection and other infectious diseases should adhere to standard precautionary principles. All patients' blood and body fluids as well as contaminated objects are considered as infectious pathogenic substances. Staff should take protective measures when they handle patients and those substances.

7.1.1 Bailing out personal protection should enacted according to the relevant requirement process when contacting patients or working in the quarantine area. This includes wearing medical protective mask, disposable cap, medical protective clothing, latex gloves, shoe covers, protective screen, goggles or any other protective gear.

7.1.2 Wearing impermeable isolating gown or waterproof apron should be done in case of blood and body fluids splash in large areas or during diagnostic and nursing procedures.

7.1.3 The medical staff whose hand skin injured should wear double gloves during diagnostic and nursing procedures that require contact with the patients' blood or body fluids.

7.1.4 Medical staff should pay attention to preventing sharp punctures or scratches by sharp instruments such as needles or suturing needles or blade during invasive diagnosis and treatment operations.

7.1.5 Sharp instruments should be placed directly into a puncture-resistant and penetrating sharp box after use. It's forbidden to directly return the needle cap and touch the sharp instruments such as needles and blades by hand after use.

7.2 In case of access the exposure risk (medical staff have had occupational exposure), it should be dealt with according to the corresponding process:

7.2.1 High exposure risk: Direct exposure to diagnosed patients including the following conditions:

ⅰ. Skin exposure: The skin is directly contaminated by a large amount of visible pollutants such as body fluids, blood, secretions or excreta of patients.

ⅱ. Mucosal exposure: The mucosal parts such as eyes or respiratory tract is directly contaminated by visible pollutants such as body fluids, blood, secretions or excreta of patients.

ⅲ. Needle stick injury: Stabs from sharp instruments contaminated with body fluids, blood, secretions or excreta of confirmed patients.

ⅳ. Direct respiratory tract exposure: Mask falls off within 1 meter of a confirmed patient without a mask leading to mouth and nose exposure.

7.2.2 Low exposure risk: Not directly exposed such as damage, detached protective gear or skin contact ,including the following conditions:

ⅰ. Broken gloves: The gloves are damaged but no direct contact of visible pollutants to the skin

ⅱ. Outer protective equipment contacts the skin or hair: The outer protective equipment comes to contact with skin or hair while taking it off.

ⅲ. Damaged protective clothing: The protective clothing is damaged but no visible pollutants directly contact the skin.

ⅳ. Indirect respiratory tract exposure: Mask fall off in front of a patient with mask or one meter away.

7.2.3 Treatment: For details, please refer to the disposal process of high-risk or low-risk exposure in the quarantine area.

7.3 Late intervention

7.3.1 Once occupational exposure occurs, report it immediately to the section head or head nurse and Leishenshan Nosocomial Infection Management Team after emergency treatment.

7.3.2 Antiviral drugs can be used for prevention under the guidance of a doctor and follow-up conducted and consultation. Monitoring of nucleic acid changes after COVID-19 exposure as well as monitoring and managing drug toxicity is important. Early related infection symptoms should be observed and recorded.

7.3.3 The Nosocomial Infection Management Team is responsible for registering occupational exposure. Registration information include: time of occupational exposure, place of exposure, the exposed site, extent of injury, type of exposure source, treatment method, treatment process, whether the preventive medication is implemented, medication compliance, regular testing and follow-up.

7.3.4 Each ward and Nosocomial Infection Management Team should regularly analyze the occupational exposure, take effective rectification measures according to the analysis results and continue to enforce occupational protection.

8. Hand Hygiene Management System

8.1 All medical staff should perform hand hygiene in strictly according to the requirements of this system. Section heads and nurses incharge need to take the lead in implementing hand hygiene practices for medical staff. Each department should conduct self-examination of hand hygiene compliance each month to improve hand hygiene compliance and accuracy.

8.2 The whole hospital must be equipped with qualified hand hygiene equipment and facilities. Packaging of hand sanitizers and dry hand items or facilities such as towels after use should in a way to avoid secondary pollution.

8.3 All medical staff must master the correct hand hygiene methods to ensure effective hand washing and disinfection.

8.4 Medical staff should correctly grasp the indications of hand wash and disinfection.

8.5 Medical staff can use quick hand disinfectants to disinfect their hands instead of washing hands when there is no visible pollutants on their hands.

8.6 Medical staff should rinse their hands with running water before disinfecting after their hands are contaminated by visible pollutants, examining, treating, taking care of infectious patients or cleaning patients' pollutants.

8.7 Hand hygiene indications

8.7.1 Before and after directly contacting patient, between contacting different patients or when moving from touching a contaminated part to a clean part of the same patient's body.

8.7.2 Before and after contact with patients' mucous membranes and damaged skin or wounds, blood, body fluids, secretions, feces or wound dressings.

8.7.3 Putting on and taking off protective equipment.

8.7.4 Before and after aseptic technique, before handling clean sterile products or after handling pollutants.

8.7.5 When the hands of medical staff are contaminated by visible pollutants, blood or body fluids

8.7.6 After touching the patients' surroundings.

9. Management System of Emergency Response Plan

9.1 Monitor and report the body temperature of hospital staff daily. Timely register the staff with respiratory and digestive suspected symptoms and keep them tracked.

9.2 For staff with abnormal body temperature and suspicious symptoms, they should be isolated in time and immediately reported to the nosocomial infection management team and the health care department. The health department will complete the relevant examinations and check the close contacts.

9.3 Implement strictly Treatment Procedure of Professional Exposure; in case of professional exposure during work, treat it in accordance to the relevant procedures.

9.4 It is strictly forbidden for any staff to conceal or misrepresent fever and respiratory symptoms in the event of professional exposure or infection. They should obey the hospital unified management and arrangement during isolation.

10. Management System of Reusable Diagnostic and Treatment Apparatus/Items

10.1 Reusable diagnostic apparatus/items in all wards of the hospital should be handled in accordance with the relevant operating procedures and specifications. They can be reused after being uniformly recycled, cleaned, disinfected/sterilized by the manufacturer. Any department or individual should not dispose them.

10.2 Reusable diagnostic apparatus/items used by patients with novel coronavirus pneumonia should be treated in accordance with the principle of disinfection–cleaning–disinfection/sterilization.

10.3 Reusable diagnostic and treatment apparatus/items in each ward should be disinfected and pretreated in the ward filth cleaning room, packaged in a double-layer Gelber Sack with wet storage, pasted with labels, and handed over to the property recovery staff.

10.4 It is recommended to use a chlorine–containing disinfectant for disinfection and pretreatment, and the effective chlorine content is 1000 mg/L.

11. Management System for Infectious Fabric

Collection of infectious fabric should be slow to avoid aerosols. Single–use fabrics should be incinerated as medical wastes. The sheets, quilts, pillowcases and other fabrics for repeated use can be sterilized by circulating steam or boiling for 30 minutes, or soaked in 500 mg/L chlorine disinfectant for 30 minutes. Cotton quilts, pillows and mattresses can be sprayed with 1000 mg/L chlorine–containing disinfectant or 500 mg/L chlorine dioxide disinfectant to moisten the surface, and then dried for 1 hour. Conditioned wards can be sterilized by bed unit sterilizers.

12. Health Management System for all Personnel

12.1 Maintaining the occupational safety of hospital staff by effectively preventing occupational hazards in all aspects of hospital work, and protecting the health of staff is a priority.

12.2 Hospital staff of all departments including medical, nursing, medical technology, pharmacy, administration and logistics are entitled to hospital medical safety.

12.3 The hospital's prevention of occupational hazards is based on occupational disease prevention laws and implementation of the prevention principles. The hospital must provide a clean working environment, reasonable work processes and necessary protective supplies for all staffs.

12.4 Strengthening the safety education for staff at work. Knowledge and skills training related to infection prevention and control, especially occupational protection training must be carried out before a staff takes up a post.

12.5 All staff are required to perform daily health monitoring, including temperature, respiratory infection symptoms, digestive tract and skin damage. Registration and follow-up should be implemented in the respective ward.

12.6 Workers should undergo regular physical examinations in accordance with relevant procedures. In case of infection or suspected infection, they should be reported and isolated for treatment as soon as possible. At the same time, follow-up investigations should be conducted on close contacts.

13. The Treatment Room Infection Management System

13.1 Non-workers are not allowed to enter. Medical personnel should wear clean clothes and hats when entering the room. Aseptic procedures and hand hygiene should be strictly implemented during operation.

13.2 Sterile and non-sterile items, cleaning items and contaminated items should be placed separately and clearly marked; the upper layer of the treatment item is the clean area and the lower layer is the contaminated area.

13.3 The room should be kept tidy. The surface of the object and the floor should be wet cleaned and disinfected twice a day. The surface of the object should be wiped with a high-level disinfection wipes. The floor should be mopped with

1000 mg/L chlorine–containing disinfectant for 30 minutes. In case of contamination, cleaning and disinfection should be done. Air disinfection should be done using air disinfection machine twice a day every one hour and recorded.

13.4 Opened sterile solution should be used within 2 hours. Once a variety of solvents, topical saline or hypertonic saline sterile cotton swabs are used, the period of use should not exceed 24 hours.

13.5 Strictly implement the management of medical waste in accordance with the relevant systems and regulations of medical waste management.

13.6 After each shift, the nurse in the treatment room should disinfect the environment and air in the treatment room.

14. Guidelines for the Use of Protective Equipment

In order to further improve the prevention and control of new COVID–19 infections at Leishenshan Hospital, effectively eliminate the risk of transmission of the new coronavirus, regulate the behavior of medical staff, combine the pathogenic characteristics of the new coronavirus, the source of infection, the route of transmission, and the susceptible population, and working characteristics of infectious disease hospitals, this guideline is specially formulated for everyone to implement. Medical institutions should take grading protection incase medical staff contact suspected or confirmed patients with new COVID–19 infection at work. Appropriate protective measures should be taken (Appendix 5). The following are the protection levels.

14.1 General protection

14.1.1 Strictly abide by the principles of standard prevention.

14.1.2 Wear work clothes and medical surgical masks when working.

14.1.3 Strictly carry out hand hygiene.

14.2 Level I protection

14.2.1 Strictly abide by the principles of standard prevention.

14.2.2 Strictly abide by the rules and regulations of disinfection and isolation.

14.2.3 Wear work clothes, isolation clothing, work caps, surgical masks, and latex gloves if necessary.

14.2.4 Strictly implement hand hygiene.

14.2.5 Perform personal hygiene when leaving the isolation area, and pay attention to the protection of the respiratory tract and mucous membrane.

14.3 Level II protection

14.3.1 Strictly abide by the principles of standard prevention.

14.3.2 Based on the route of transmission, take droplet isolation and contact isolation.

14.3.3 Strictly abide by the rules and regulations of disinfection and isolation.

14.3.4 Medical personnel entering the isolation ward and isolation ward must wear medical protective masks, work clothes, isolation clothing and/or medical protective clothing, shoe covers, gloves, work caps, and goggles or protective screens if necessary. Strictly accordance with the division of clean area, potential pollution area and pollution area, wear and remove protective equipment properly. Pay close attention to oral cavity, nasal mucosa and eye conjunctiva hygiene and protection.

14.4 Level III protection

The tertiary protection is based on the secondary protection, fortify a positive pressure headgear or a comprehensive respiratory protective device.

15. Emergency Plan for Controlling Outbreaks of Infection in Wuhan Leishenshan Hospital

15.1 Object

In order to prevent, control and eliminate the outbreak and serious consequences of nosocomial infection, guide and standardize the emergency treatment of nosocomial infection outbreak and protect the health of patients and medical staff, this plan is formulated by regulations such as the *Law of the People's Republic of China on the prevention and treatment of infectious diseases, Emergency Regulations for Public Health Emergencies, Regulations on public health emergencies, Code for the Management of Reporting and Disposal of Nosocomial Infection, Code for the Monitoring of Nosocomial Infection*, as well as other laws and regulations in combination with the actual situation in Leishenshan Hospital.

15.2 Range of application

This plan applies to emergency treatment in case of outbreaks or suspected outbreak of nosocomial infection in Wuhan Leishenshan Hospital.

15.3 Definition and classification of nosocomial infection outbreak

15.3.1 Definition

ⅰ.Nosocomial infection outbreak: refers to the occurrence of more than 3 cases of homologous infection in a short period of time among patients in a medical institution or department.

ⅱ.Suspected outbreak of nosocomial infection: refers to the occurrence of more than 3 cases with similar clinical symptoms and suspected common infection source, or more than 3 cases with suspected common infection source or infection pathway in a short period of time among patients in a medical institution or department.

15.3.2 Classification

ⅰ.Grade Ⅰ : more than 10 cases of nosocomial infection outbreak; nosocomial infection with special pathogens or new pathogens; nosocomial infection that may cause significant public effect or serious consequences.

ⅱ.Grade Ⅱ : more than 5 cases of nosocomial infection outbreaks; death directly caused by nosocomial infection outbreak; more than 3 cases of personal injury caused by nosocomial infection outbreak.

ⅲ.Grade Ⅲ : More than 3 cases of nosocomial infection outbreaks or more than 5 cases of suspected outbreaks of nosocomial infections.

15.4 Emergency organization and responsibilities

Leishenshan Hospital set up a leading group for emergency response to nosocomial infection. The leading group has an emergency office. Its responsibilities and tasks are as follows:

15.4.1 Leading group of nosocomial infection outbreak

ⅰ. Responsibility: Leading group investigates and formulates control plans for nosocomial infection outbreak. When there is epidemic or nosocomial infection outbreaks, the group would be responsible for making final judgments on the establishment of nosocomial infection outbreak. It would also coordinate related departments to carry out investigation and control the outbreak. They are then required to report to the relevant health administrative departments.

ⅱ. Staffing:

Group leader: one

Deputy leader: several

Group member: several (including each medical team head)

15.4.2 Emergency Nosocomial Infection Outbreak Disposal Office (attached to the Quality Management Institute of Medical Management Department)

ⅰ. Responsibility: This office is specifically responsible for implementing the resolutions of the leading group, advising hospital to work in accordance with the emergency plan, confirming the implementation of various disposal measures, and coordinating the supervision of information reports, notifications, and epidemic reporting, etc. The clinical medical technology, administrative and logistical support departments of the hospital must obey the unified coordination and guidelines of the office for prevention of public health emergencies.

ⅱ. Staffing: Office manager: one

Office member: several (including the person responsible of infection prevention and control in each medical team)

Secretary: one

15.5 Surveillance and reporting of nosocomial infection

15.5.1 Each ward should proactively monitor outbreak of nosocomial infection according to the general requirements of the hospital. The Emergency Management Office strengthens the management and supervision of the surveillance quality as follows:

ⅰ. The hospital establishes a monitoring and feedback network trinity consisting of nosocomial infection management team, clinical laboratory department and nosocomial infection management team in each ward to improve the emergency response capacity for detection and monitoring of suspected nosocomial infection outbreak.

ⅱ. Perfect nosocomial infection case consultation system: When an outbreak of nosocomial infection is established and consultation or verification of the infection is needed, the medical team would be responsible for contacting relevant experts to complete the consultation or verify the diagnosis.

15.5.2 In every ward, one of the following instances should be reported to the nosocomial infection management team immediately (can be reported to the person on duty in case its non–working time).

ⅰ. The doctor in charge and the nurse responsible for nosocomial infection control finds more than 3 cases of the same pathogen infection within a short period of time in the department. The doctor in charge should initially judge whether it is nosocomial infection outbreak. If the judgement is "yes" or "highly suspect", he/she should immediately report to the director of the department. The director will check the above cases and if confirmed they should immediately report to the nosocomial infection management team.

ⅱ. If surveillance personnel from the nosocomial infection management team and ward management staff find more than 3 nosocomial infection cases with the same syndrome in the same department within a short period of time, they should immediately do epidemiological investigation and report to infection management committee.

ⅲ. The content of the report is divided into the first report, the process report and the case closing report according to the regulations of the national and provincial health administration departments. The event process is timely reported according to the severity of the incident, the development of the situation and the control situation.

ⅳ. No department or individual should instruct others to or directly conceal, postpone or misrepresent the incident of nosocomial infection.

15.6 Notification on nosocomial infection outbreak information

15.6.1 The nosocomial infection management team must report to the Jiangxia District Health Administration Department and Jiangxia District Center for

Disease Control and Prevention within 12 hours according to the provisions of the *Nosocomial Infection Outbreak Report and Disposal Management Regulations* upon investigation and verification of the following situations:

ⅰ. More than 5 suspected cases of nosocomial infection.

ⅱ. More than 3 cases of nosocomial infection.

15.6.2 Hospital must report to the Jiangxia District Health Administration Department and the Jiangxia District Center for Disease Control and Prevention within 2 hours in accordance with the requirements of the *National Standards for the Management of Public Health Emergency Related Information Reports (Trial)* under the following circumstances:

ⅰ. More than 10 cases of nosocomial infection outbreak.

ⅱ. Nosocomial infection with special or new pathogens.

ⅲ. Nosocomial infection that may cause significant public effect or serious consequences.

15.7 Emergency response and end of nosocomial infection outbreak

15.7.1 Emergency response in case of nosocomial infection outbreak

ⅰ. When there is a trend of nosocomial infection outbreak or when an outbreak is confirmed in the clinical department, concerned personnel should immediately report to the medical management department and the nosocomial infection management team. After receiving the notification, the nosocomial infection management team should go to the ward immediately to check and confirm the situation. Upon the initial confirmation of nosocomial infection outbreak, he/she should report to the leadership of the hospital and related departments, and then initiate a preplan.

ⅱ. The emergency leadership team of nosocomial infection outbreak should promptly consolidate relevant departments to cooperate with the nosocomial infection management team to carry out epidemiological investigation and disposition of infection outbreak, guarantee human, material and financial resources.

ⅲ. Infection prevention and emergency control treatment experts are responsible for infection prevention, control, and treatment under the unified arrangement of emergency leadership team of nosocomial infection outbreak.

ⅳ. The nosocomial infection management team strengthens the surveillance of the epidemic and closely follows the epidemic situation under the supervision of the emergency leadership group.

ⅴ. Emergency leadership team of nosocomial infection outbreak performs inspection and supervision of various specific tasks, and adopts measures such as disinfection and isolation to prevent curb epidemic outbreak.

ⅵ. All related departments should strictly complete patient diagnosis and treatment, disinfection and isolation of medical treatment areas, and personal protection of medical personnel.

ⅶ. Publicity department should promote health education.

ⅷ. The hospital finance, equipment, and pharmacy departments should provide emergency fund, material and drugs support in time in accordance with the requirements of the emergency leadership team of nosocomial infection.

ⅸ. Responsibilities of relevant departments in emergency response

ⅰ) Duties of each clinical department

① When the department discovers sporadic cases of nosocomial infection, they should timely report through the monitoring information software of nosocomial infection within 24 hours. When they discover a trend of nosocomial infection outbreak, the department must immediately report to the nosocomial infection management team.

② Each department should promptly arrange for physician consultation from the infection department in case of a suspicious case.

③ Each department should arrange for pathogenic tests and drug sensitivity tests in time to find the source and route of infection. Each department should actively treat their patients and control the spread of nosocomial infection.

④ The infection management team of each department should timely mobilize to find the cause of nosocomial infection and report to the nosocomial infection management team.

⑤ Each department should actively work with others to complete epidemiological investigations, carefully formulate and implement control measures of nosocomial infection. If the nosocomial infection is diagnosed as an infectious disease, the department should report in accordance with the requirements of the *Law of Infectious Disease Prevention and Control* and the *Infectious Disease Information Reporting Management Regulations*.

⑥ Each department should organize nurses to implement group care and restrict transfer of the patients in or out if necessary.

⑦ The principles for the placement of hospital-infected patients should be as follows: infected patients should be separated from non-infected patients, patients with the same type of infection should be concentrated in one place. Patients with special infection disease should be placed in accordance with the *Law on the Prevention and Treatment of Infectious Diseases*.

⑧ The concept of hand hygiene should be strengthened, disinfection measures strictly implemented, and medical staff educated and trained on knowledge and skills of nosocomial infection prevention and control.

ⅱ) Responsibilities of QC team:

① Immediately organize full-time staff to conduct epidemiological investigation, and coordinate with clinical departments to carefully collect epidemiological data.

② Search for the source of infection: etiological investigation should be carried out on infected patients, contacts, suspected sources of infection, environment, articles, medical staff and accompanying personnel. Microbiological data should be carefully collected.

③ Confirmation of the outbreak of nosocomial infection: for the similar infection cases suspected to occur in the same period, experts from the infection department should be consulted to verify the diagnosis in time, and confirm whether there is an outbreak of nosocomial infection according to the regulations of *Nosocomial infection outbreak report and disposal Management Standard*. At the same time, this should be reported to the director in charge, the medical team, nursing team, the pharmacy department and cleaning department to assist in the investigation.

④ Consult within the department to formulate corresponding control measures. To guide and supervise the infection control measures in the department:

a. The patients suspected of outbreaks or outbreaks are centrally isolated. Grouped nursing, restricted visits, and personal protection of medical staff are strengthened. Surfaces disinfected with 1000 mg/L chlorin three times a daily, i.e. once in the morning, once in the afternoon and once in the evening. If the outbreak is still uncontrolled after centralized isolation, measures such as suspending the admission of new patients are considered.

b. Strengthen the implementation of hand hygiene and aseptic technical operation.

c. Rational use of anti-infective drugs to control the use of some special antimicrobials.

d. Strengthen the cleaning and disinfection of reusable diagnosis and treatment instruments.

e. To protect susceptible patients, in case of infectious nosocomial infections, they must be managed in accordance with the relevant provisions of the *Infectious Diseases Prevention and Treatment Law.*

f. If you encounter difficult problems in epidemiological investigation and emergency response, you should consult the expert group in time.

g. Analyze the investigation data, describe in details the distribution of the department, population and time of the cases. Analyze the causes of the outbreak, and speculate the possible source of infection, route of infection or susceptible factors. Combine these with results of laboratory examination and the effect of control measures to make a preliminary evaluation.

h. Organize full-time staff to monitor the cases of nosocomial infection, observe the incidence of new cases, and evaluate the effect in time.

i. Write an investigation report, sum up experience and formulate preventive measures.

J Strengthen publicity and education, organize medical staff to train on the knowledge of nosocomial infection to improve their ability to monitor and implement sensory control intervention measures.

ⅲ) Responsibilities of the medical team:

① When there is an outbreak trend of nosocomial infection, coordinate the nosocomial infection management team to organize relevant departments to carry out nosocomial infection investigation and control. According to the needs, deploy the doctors. Timely organize the treatment and aftercare of patients as well as the dispatch of drugs and equipment.

② When the outbreak trend of nosocomial infection requires consultation or verification of diagnosis of infected cases, the Ministry of Medical Education is responsible for organizing relevant experts to complete the task of case consultation or verification of diagnosis. Jointly, they should formulate relevant control measures to guide and supervise the departmental implementations.

ⅳ) Responsibilities of the nursing team:

When there is an outbreak of nosocomial infection, the nursing human resources should be assigned according to the needs. The disinfection and isolation measures should be strictly carried out, and the special cases of nosocomial infection should be nursed separately if necessary.

ⅴ) Responsibilities of the infection expert group:

① Accept the arrangement of the hospital to actively participate in the consultation of nosocomial infection cases and guide departments to make rational use of antibiotics.

② Instruct the QC team to complete the epidemiological investigation in time and jointly formulate control measures to curb the situation.

ⅵ) Responsibilities of the Nosocomial Infection Committee:

① Timely convene a meeting of the committee on the *management of nosocomial infection* to assess the outbreak trend and decide whether to start or terminate the emergency plan.

② Timely organize relevant departments to provide human, material and financial support to control the outbreak of nosocomial infection in time.

③ Advise the nosocomial infection management team to report the outbreak of nosocomial infection in accordance with the provisions of the measures for the Management of Nosocomial Infection.

15.7.2 The end of nosocomial infection outbreak:

The end of the outbreak of nosocomial infection should meet the following conditions: after the concealed risk or related risk factors of the outbreak of nosocomial infection are eliminated, or when there were no new cases after the last case of nosocomial infection. Whether to end it or not is decided by experts chosen by the emergency leading group for the outbreak of nosocomial infection.

15.7.3 Late evaluation of nosocomial infection outbreaks:

After completion of the emergency treatment of nosocomial infection outbreaks, the Nosocomial Infection Management Committee should evaluate handling of emergencies. The evaluation mainly includes the state of the incident, the state of on–the–spot investigation and treatment, the treatment of patients, evaluation of the of the measures taken, the existing problems in the course of emergency treatment, the experience gained and recommendations for improvement. The evaluation report should be reported to the hospital leaders and/or relevant superior departments based on level of the incident.

15.8. Emergency protection of nosocomial infection outbreaks

15.8.1 Personnel support:

ⅰ) To set up an expert group for emergency control of nosocomial infection outbreaks.

① To be responsible for technical guidance on health emergency treatment of nosocomial infection outbreaks; to carry out medical treatment of infection cases and put forward proposals on the next step of prevention and control measures; supervise and manage the safety protection work in the course of emergency handling, and guide nosocomial infection outbreak epidemiological investigations; to guide the sample collection, transportation and pathogen detection during outbreaks.

② Team leader: one,

Deputy leader: two

Member: several

ii) Set up a nosocomial infection outbreak emergency medical team.

iii) According to the situation of the outbreak, the personnel above the attending physician are transferred to the relevant departments to form an emergency prevention and control team. They participate in the treatment of the outbreak, the prevention and control of the epidemic at any time.

15.8.2 Professional training of technical personnel related to technical support and emergency medical teams should include regular training and drills to continuously improve the level of emergency treatment.

15.8.3 Material support from hospital materials department, pharmacy department, etc., should have a certain reserve base for emergency materials (emergency equipment, disinfection drugs, testing reagents, special drugs, etc.).

15.8.4 Fund guarantee the emergency leading group for the outbreak of nosocomial infection plans to reserve a certain amount of special health fund according to the actual situation of the hospital.

16. Emergency Plan for Loss, Leakage, Diffusion and Accidents during Medical Waste Handling at Wuhan Leishenshan Hospital

16.1 Purpose

In order to deal with emergencies such as the loss, leakage, spread and accident of medical waste in our hospital, the following emergency plan is specifically formulated.

16.2 Main content

16.2.1 All the staff members of the hospital are responsible for reporting immediately to the supervision or expert departments such as the Hospital-Acquired Infection Control Department, the Logistics Support Department, the Medical Management Department in case of medical waste loss, leakage, spread, and accidents. Relevant departments of the hospital should immediately consolidate manpower to identify the cause and formulate preventive measures.

16.2.2 If serious incidents such as medical waste overflow, scattered or truck overturning, worker injury occur during medical waste transportation, the person in charge or the accident department should immediately report to the relevant departments such as the Logistics Support Department or Hospital–Acquired Infection Control Department.

16.2.3 After receiving the call, the staff of the relevant departments should immediately rush to the scene of medical waste leakage and diffusion to assist the parties concerned or the personnel of the accident department to complete emergency treatment measures.

16.2.4 The security team is responsible for establishing a quarantine area for the medical waste leakage and diffusion site. They should restrict other vehicles and pedestrians from accessing the site to prevent the spread of pollutants and harm.

16.2.5 The staff of the relevant departments, such as the Logistics Support Department and the Hospital–Acquired Infection Control Department should work with the concerned personnel to determine the type, quantity, time of occurrence, scope and severity of the medical waste that was lost, leaked, and diffused. They should also assist in investigating the cause of the accident.

16.2.6 The relevant personnel of the Logistics Support Department are responsible for the rapid collection, cleaning and disinfection of spilled and scattered medical waste. Clean–up personnel should wear protective clothing, gloves, masks, boots and other protective equipment when carrying out the cleaning work. After the cleaning work is completed, appliances and protective equipment must be disinfected.

16.2.7 The Hospital–Acquired Infection Control Department is responsible for supervising the treatment of medical waste contaminated areas. The process should minimize effect on patients, medical staff, other on–site personnel as well as the environment.

16.2.8 When disinfecting areas contaminated with infectious waste, disinfection is carried out from the least polluted areas to the most polluted areas. All the tools used that may be contaminated should be disinfected. The effect on patients, medical personnel, other on–site personnel and the environment should be minimized.

16.2.9 If the body (skin) of the cleaning staff is accidentally contaminated, the contaminated area should be flushed with water in the vicinity. If accidentally injured, they should be promptly treated in the nearest consultation room.

16.2.10 When medical waste is lost at a medical waste staging point, it shall be reported to the Logistics Support Department and the Hospital-Acquired Infection Control Department, and the hospital supervisor leadership level by level. The lost medical waste should be recovered as soon as possible.

16.2.11 In the event of medical waste loss, leakage, diffusion and accidents, corresponding emergency measures should be taken in accordance with the provisions of The Medical Waste Management Regulations and The Medical Waste Management Measures of Medical Institutions. It should be reported to the Jiangxia District Health Commission and the Environmental Protection Bureau within 48 hours. After investigation and processing, the results should be reported to the Jiangxia District Health Commission and the Environmental Protection Bureau

16.2.12 In case of a major accident where medical aid and on-site rescue are required to be provided to the injured persons, death of more than 1 person or health impairment of more than 3 people due to improper management of the medical waste, it should be reported to the Jiangxia District Health Commission and the Environmental Protection Bureau within 12 hours. Appropriate emergency treatment measures should be taken in accordance with the Medical Waste Management Regulations and the Medical Waste Management Measures of Medical Institutions.

16.2.13 In the event of a major accident where medical aid and on-site rescue are required to be provided to the sick person due to improper management of medical waste leading to the death of more than 3 person or health harm in more than 10 people, it should be reported to the Jiangxia District Health Commission and the Environmental Protection Bureau within 2 hours. Eventually, appropriate emergency treatment measures should be taken in accordance with the Medical Waste Management Regulations and the Medical Waste Management Measures of Medical Institutions.

16.2.14 When an infectious disease transmission accident occurs due to improper management of medical waste, or there is evidence of likelihood of an accident, it should be reported in accordance with the *Law on the Prevention and Control of Infectious Diseases*. Eventually, the relevant provisions and corresponding measures should be taken.

16.2.15 After the treatment is completed, the Hospital Management Leading Group for Medical Waste must organize an investigation on the cause of the incident and take effective precautions to prevent a similar incident.

16.2.16 The Logistics Support Department should enhance training of cleaning company workers and medical waste transport workers on the management of medical waste disposal, and strict prevention of loss, leakage, spread and accidents.

16.2.17 The Hospital–Acquired Infection Control Department should check the implementation of the medical waste management measures throughout the hospital on a monthly basis and incorporate the results of the inspection results into the quality assessment of the departments.

17. High Temperature and Heatstroke Prevention Emergency Plan

17.1 Purpose

Summer in Wuhan area comes relatively early and around March the average temperature can reach about 24 degrees. In view of the fact that during the epidemic, the staff of Wuhan Leishenshan Hospital wore protective equipment, it further aggravated the body temperature and the risk of high temperature heatstroke heightened. To prevent heatstroke in the personnel working in the high–temperature climate environment, to ensure the smooth progress of various medical work, fast and effective response to emergency rescue a special plan is formulated.

17.2 Scope of application

This plan applies to all staff in the hospital. The key prevention personnel (project management offices) are: the isolation ward staff and peripheral support staff.

17.3 Main content

17.3.1 The Hospital–Acquired Infection Control Department should carry out various forms of extensive publicity on the prevention and treatment of heatstroke in advance before the summer. This will help the staff to master the basic information on heatstroke prevention and cooling, as well as understand the physical reaction before heatstroke.

17.3.2 The Logistics Support Department should strengthen the management of hydropower supply for all projects in summer to ensure availability of electricity and water in the wards. In case of special circumstances requiring power outages and water outages, the relevant departments should be notified in advance and corresponding adjustments should be made.

17.3.3 The Logistics Support Department should purchase a batch of cooling chemicals in advance, and distribute the heatstroke cooling items to each ward and each working group as required. They may also distribute heatstroke cooling drinks according to the real-time condition.

17.3.4 The Health Section of the Medical Group should improve understanding of the physical condition to the medical personnel in the event of heatstroke such as syncope and dehydration.

17.3.5 According to the high temperature situation and the working conditions of medical personnel in the ward, the Hospital-Acquired Infection Control Department and the Medical Team recommended these measures: shorten the working time in the isolation ward, focus your time on peripheral support work, use heatstroke cooling drinks, and place water dispensers in clean areas .

17.3.6 Mild heatstroke staff: When the staff feels dizzy, fatigued, and dazzled during normal work, they should immediately stop working to prevent secondary heat stroke. Those with mild heatstroke in the isolation ward, should quickly take off protective equipment in a separate room under the assistance of other personnel and quickly evacuate the isolation room. They should take use of cold water, medicine, wet towels, etc. in a clean area.

17.3.7 Severe heatstroke staff (fainted, shocked, severely dehydrated, etc.): When the staff suffer from heatstroke, close personnel should immediately take them to a cool and ventilated area to observe their symptoms for first-hand medical information to medical personnel. Subsequently, they should notify the Medical office and the Hospital–Acquired Infection Control Department. This will organize rescue workers in the first time to transfer heatstroke patients to the nearest hospital for observation, treatment, and report to the company's branch leader.

　　17.3.8 During treatment and after the treatment of the employees suffering from heatstroke, the relevant personnel is required to pay more attention to the physical condition of the employees and calm their emotions. They should encourage them to receive treatment with peace of mind and assure them they can work again once their physical strength is fully restored.

Part 2   Standard Operating Procedures

1. The Process of Wearing Medical Disposable Surgical Mask

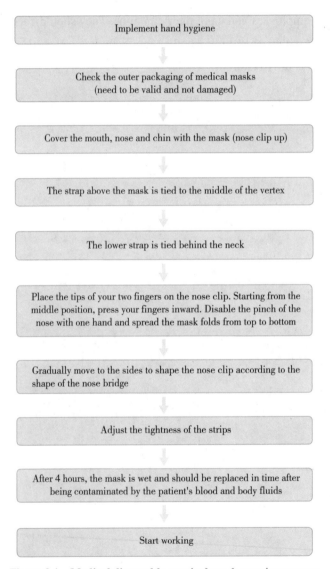

Figure 3.1   Medical disposable surgical mask wearing process

2. The Process of Wearing Medical Particulate Respirator

Implement hand hygiene

↓

Check the outer packaging of medical particulate respirator
(need to be valid and not damaged)

↓

Hold the medical particulate respirator with one hand
(the side with the nose clip facing out and up)

↓

Cover nose, mouth and chin with medical particulate respirator

↓

Pull the lower strap over your head with the other hand and place it on your neck

↓

Then pull the top strap to the middle of the head

↓

Place both index fingers on the metal nose clip→Start from the middle
with one hand pressing the inward→Move and press from both sides,
respectively→Shape the clip according to the bridge of the nose

↓

Inspect for tightness
(Method: breathe quickly with both hands covered with medical
particulate respirator)

↓   ↓

Air leak near the nose clip   Air leak is around

↓

Adjust to air tight

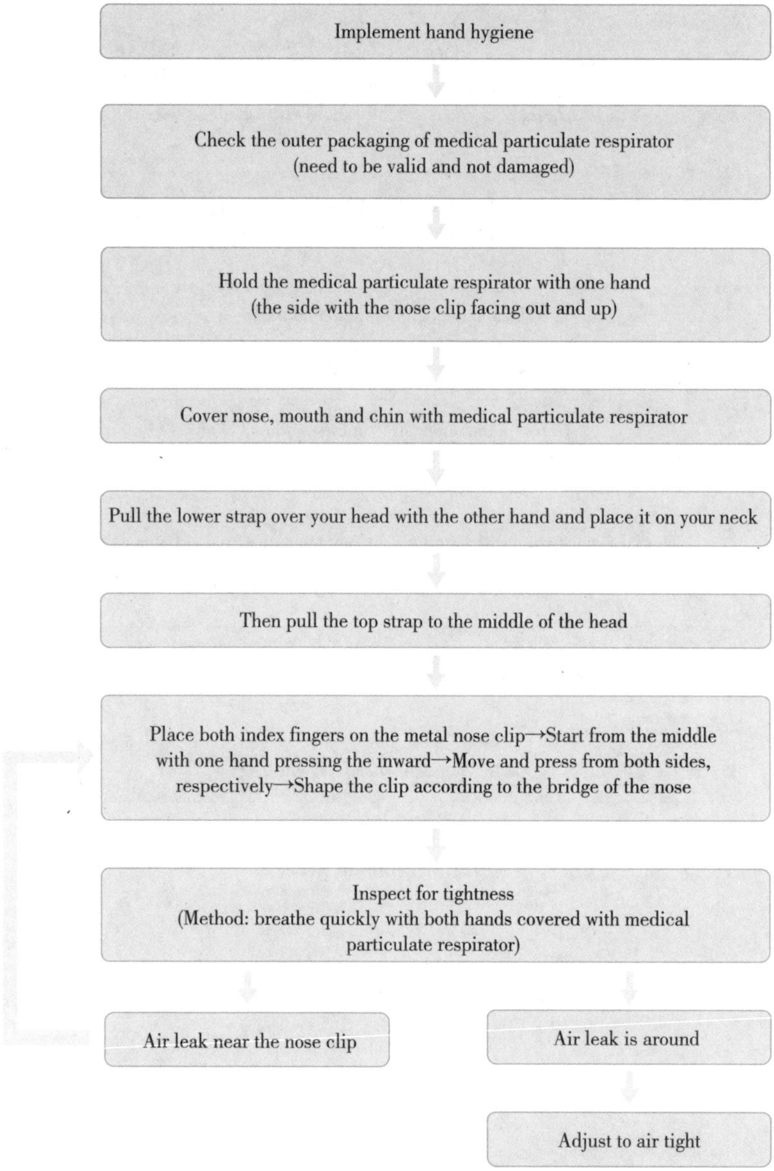

Figure 3.2   Medical particulate respirator wearing process

3. The Process of Removing Medical Disposable Surgical Mask,
Medical Particulate Respirator

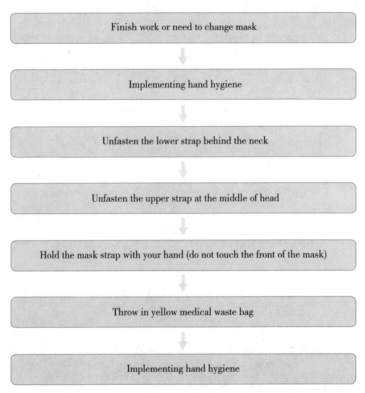

Figure 3.3   Medical disposable surgical mask, medical particulate
respirator removal process

4. The Standard Operation Procedure of Wearing Protective Equipment for Quarantine Staff

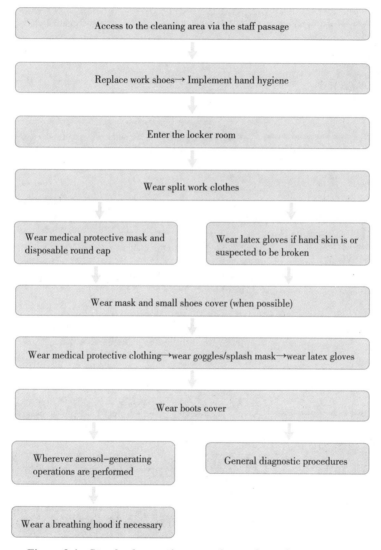

Figure 3.4 Standard operation procedures of wearing protective equipment for quarantine staff

5. The Standard Operation Procedure of Taking off Protective Equipment for Quarantine Staff

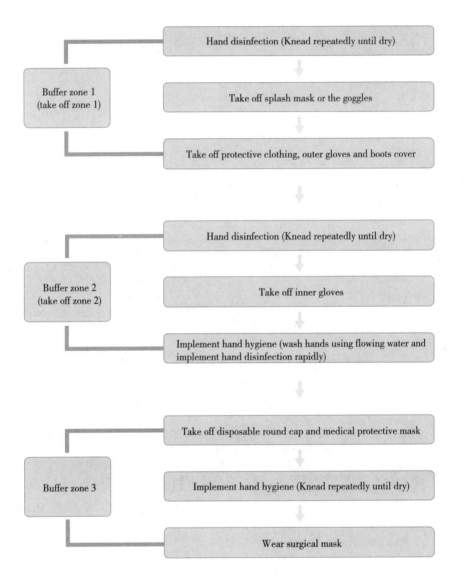

*The above regional arrangements are set according to the architectural characteristics of Leishenshan Hospital

Figure 3.5   Standard operation procedure of removing protective equipment for
quarantine staff

6. The Standard Operation Procedure of Wearing Medical Protective Clothing for Quarantine Staff

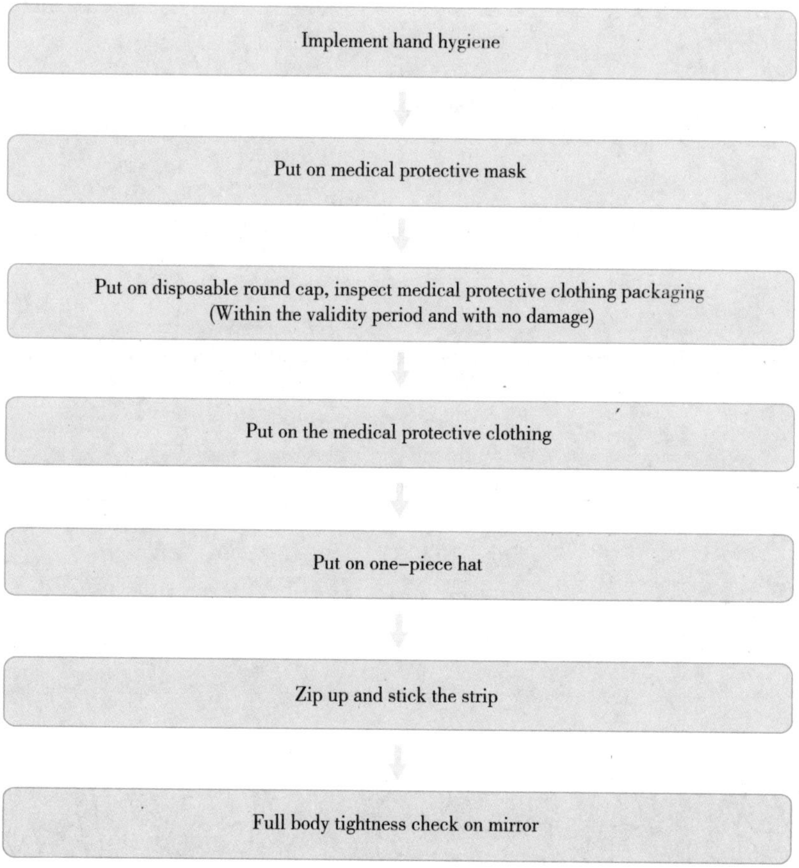

Implement hand hygiene

↓

Put on medical protective mask

↓

Put on disposable round cap, inspect medical protective clothing packaging
(Within the validity period and with no damage)

↓

Put on the medical protective clothing

↓

Put on one-piece hat

↓

Zip up and stick the strip

↓

Full body tightness check on mirror

Figure 3.6   Standard operation procedure of wearing medical protective
clothing for staff at quarantine centers

7. Procedures of Removing Overall Medical Protective Clothing for Staff

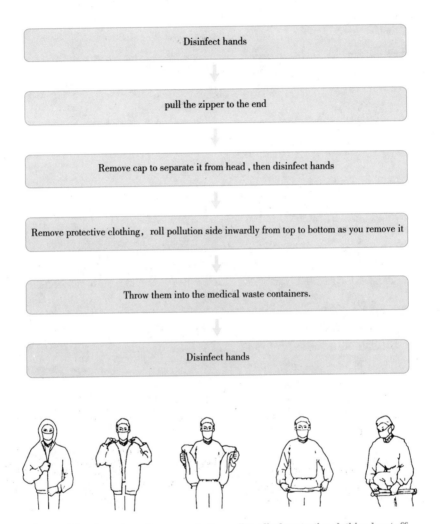

Disinfect hands

pull the zipper to the end

Remove cap to separate it from head , then disinfect hands

Remove protective clothing, roll pollution side inwardly from top to bottom as you remove it

Throw them into the medical waste containers.

Disinfect hands

Figure 3.7   Procedures for removal of overall medical protective clothing by staff

8. Cleaning and Disinfecting Procedures of the Ward

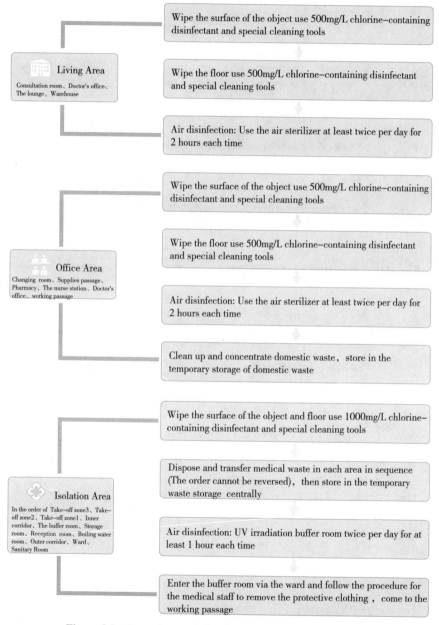

Figure 3.8   Procedures of cleaning and disinfection of wards

9. Terminal Disinfection Procedures of the Bed Unit

Patient discharged

↓

Cleaning staff wear protective equipment

↓

Remove sheets, bedding covers, pillowcases and other cotton supplies

↓

Dispose them as medical waste ,   put in yellow garbage bag

↓

Wipe and disinfect all object surfaces and floors, use the bed unit sterilizer to disinfect the bed unit

↓

When the room is unoccupied, use hydrogen peroxide air sterilizer for room air disinfection

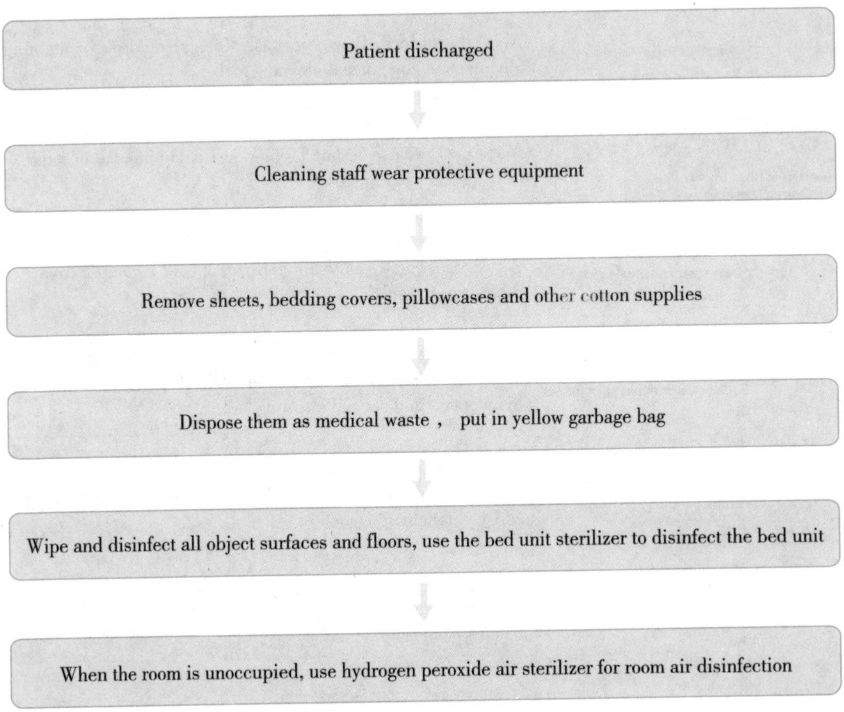

Figure 3.9   Terminal disinfection procedures of the bed unit

10. The Process Examining outpatients in the Isolation Areas

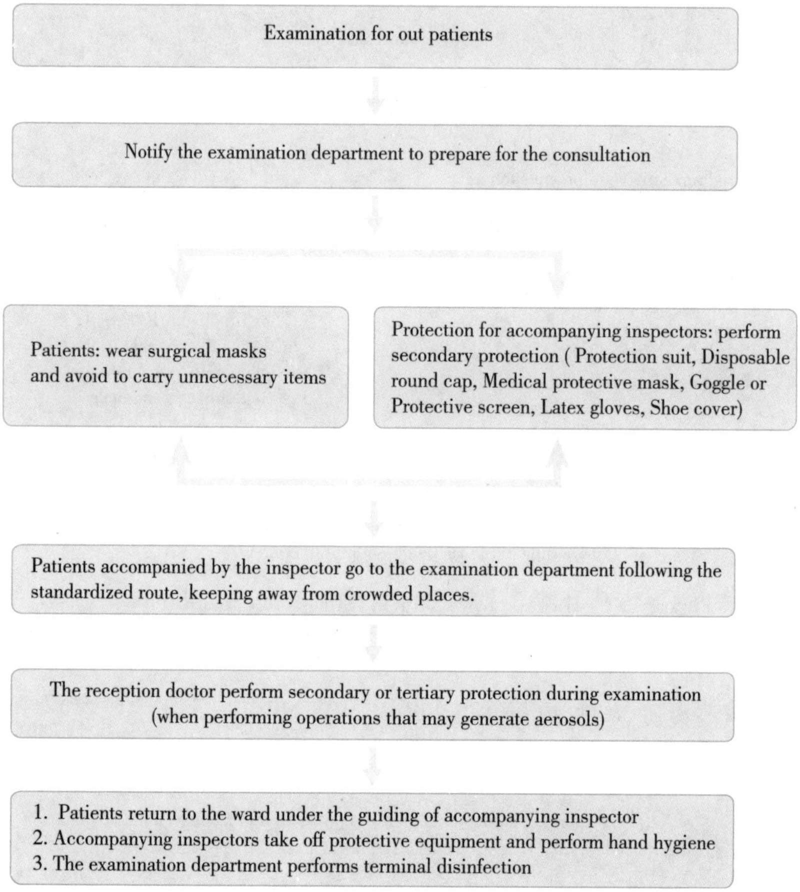

Examination for out patients

Notify the examination department to prepare for the consultation

Patients: wear surgical masks and avoid to carry unnecessary items

Protection for accompanying inspectors: perform secondary protection (Protection suit, Disposable round cap, Medical protective mask, Goggle or Protective screen, Latex gloves, Shoe cover)

Patients accompanied by the inspector go to the examination department following the standardized route, keeping away from crowded places.

The reception doctor perform secondary or tertiary protection during examination (when performing operations that may generate aerosols)

1. Patients return to the ward under the guiding of accompanying inspector
2. Accompanying inspectors take off protective equipment and perform hand hygiene
3. The examination department performs terminal disinfection

Figure 3.10   Examination process for out-patients in isolation areas

11. Handling Process of Reusable Medical Devices

```
                    Medical devices after use

Personal protective equipment such as      Other reusable medical devices
goggles that need to be reused

Putting into the soaking box          Transporting to the soaking
filled with 1000mg/L chlorine         box filled with 1000mg/L
disinfectant in the buffer room       chlorine disinfectant in the
for taking off protective devices     contaminated room through
                                      contaminated channels

        Packaging by double yellow medical waste bag and
        transporting to the Disinfection Supply Center
```

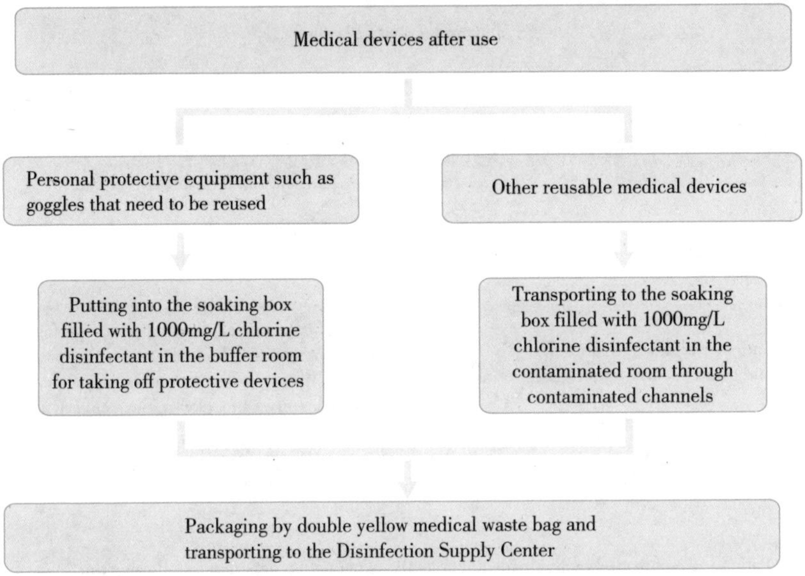

Figure 3.11　Handling procedures for reusable medical devices

12. Process of Cleaning and Disinfecting Sample Transfer Box

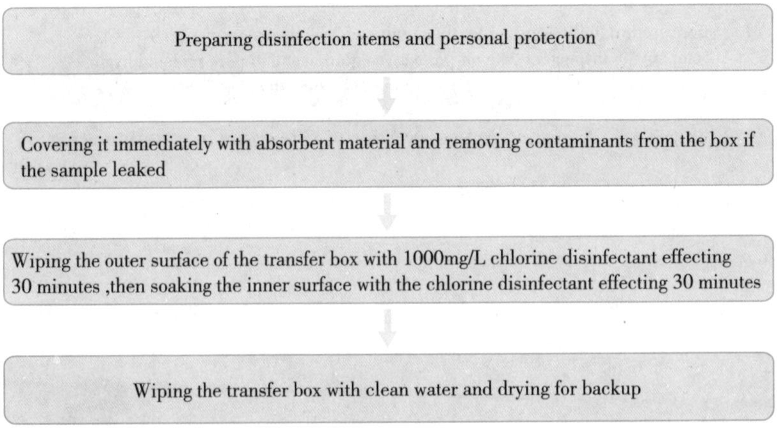

```
        Preparing disinfection items and personal protection

Covering it immediately with absorbent material and removing contaminants from the box if
the sample leaked

Wiping the outer surface of the transfer box with 1000mg/L chlorine disinfectant effecting
30 minutes ,then soaking the inner surface with the chlorine disinfectant effecting 30 minutes

        Wiping the transfer box with clean water and drying for backup
```

Figure 3.12　Cleaning and disinfection procedures of sample transfer box

13. Medical Waste Collection and Transfer Flow Chart

Hospital waste

Non-medical waste (Wastes generated mainly from clean areas such as administrative regions, doctor or nurse's rooms)	Medical waste (Wastes generated mainly from each wards, treatment rooms, laboratory department; domestic rubbish of patients or patients with NCP; areas suspects have touched or affected regions

Package with black garbage bag

Infectious	Pathological	Chemical	Pharmaceutical	Hazardous

Pack hermetically

Package with Gelber Sack	Sharps container

Send it to the temporary storage of domestic garbage and make a record

No more than 3/4

Sealed double-layer package:Gooseneck layered package sealing with cable tie

Labelling:include generating hospital,department,date,category(Mark "Novel coronavirus"),weight.

Handover and signature:the ward and the transfer personnel weigh and hand over and both sign to keep

Out of handover:add a layer of Gerbel Sack or spray with disinfectant

Attention:If the packaging bag or sharps box is contaminated, add a layer of garbage bag on the outside. It is forbidden to squeeze the protective clothing and other items in the bag to avoid the generation of aerosols.

Send it to city garbage disposal center

Clean the temporary storage place and transportation tools in time after each cleaning

Transit according to the designated route, and cannot be mixed with domestic garbage

Send medical waste to temporary storage and make handover records

Send to medical waste incineration station for centralized disposal.All transfer records need to be kept for three years

At the end of each day's delivery, the delivery tool is sterilized with 1000mg / L chlorine-containing disinfectant. When transportation tools are contaminated, disinfect at any time. Use 1000mg / L chlorine disinfectant to disinfect the ground of the medical waste storage place twice a day.

Figure 3.13   Procedure of medical waste collection and transfer

14. Preparation Process of Disinfection Liquid

Personal protection(Gloves + Mask + Cap)

↓

Prepare related items(Graduated container,disinfectant and test paper)

↓

Prepare solution according to the required concentration of daily cleaning and disinfection regulations in the ward

↓

After dissolution, determine the effective concentration with the residual chlorine concentration test paper

Figure 3.14　Preparation process of disinfection liquid

15.The Process of Disposal of Remains from Patients with Novel Coronavirus Pneumonia

> After the death of the patient, the hospital reports to the health and administrative department at the corresponding level

> Personal protection:Wear work clothes, disposable work caps, disposable gloves and long–sleeved thick latex gloves, medical disposable protective clothing, KN95 / N95 or above particulate protective masks or medical protective masks, work shoes or rubber boots, waterproof boot covers, waterproof apron or waterproof isolation gown, etc.

> Use 3000 ~ 5000mg / L chlorine–containing disinfectant or 0.5% peracetic acid cotton ball or gauzeto fill all open channels or wounds such as the patient's mouth, nose, ears, anus, tracheotomy.Wrap the body with a double–layer cloth impregnated with chlorine–containing disinfectant, and put it in a double–layer corpse bag to seal it. Never open it after sealing

> Handover to the funeral home

> Terminal disinfection of remains disposal area
> Air disinfection:spray with 3% hydrogen peroxide
> Object surface disinfection:wipe the surface of the object with 2000mg / L chlorine–containing disinfectant for 30 minutes
> Dispose of contaminated clothing, etc. as medical waste

> Take off personal protective equipment and do the hand hygiene

Figure 3.15   Disposal procedure for the remains of patients with novel coronavirus

16.The Process of Infection Prevention/Control for Discharged Patients

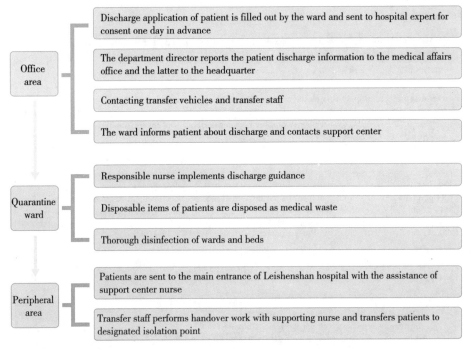

Figure 3.16   Process of infection prevention/control for discharged patients

17. Emergency Handling Procedure of Damaged Protective Clothing

Accidental damage of protective clothing in the quarantine area

↓

Pinching the surrounding area of the damage as soon as possible

↓

Sticking the damaged area with tape at the same time

↓

Entering the first area of taking off the protective clothing and disinfecting hands

↓

Taking off the outer gloves and disinfecting hands

↓

Spraying chlorine–containing disinfectant (1000 mg/L) on damaged area

↓

Taking off the protective clothing and disinfecting hands

↓

Spraying chlorine–containing disinfectant (1000mg/L) on the inner layer corresponding to the damaged area

↓

Completing the process of removing protective gear

↓

Re–wearing protective equipment and entering the quarantine area

↓

Reporting to the infection control staff and department director in time, scanning QR code and reporting occupational exposure

Figure 3.17   Emergency handling procedure for damaged protective clothing

18. Emergency Handling Procedure of Staff in Quarantine Ward Who
Abruptly become Unconscious

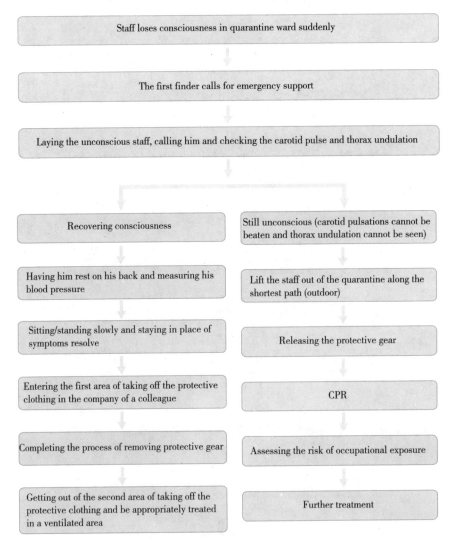

Figure 3.18   Emergency handling procedure for staff in quarantine wards who
suddenly become unconscious

19. Syncope Emergency Treatment Process in the Isolation Area

Prodromal symptoms appear and do not disappear quickly (such as persistent nausea, sweating, chest tightness, palpitation, awareness of defecation, etc.)

↓

Inform colleagues in the quarantine area and suspend work

↓

Sit or lie flat in a relatively clean area and inhale oxygen as appropriate

↓

Choose the appropriate PCM action

↓

Measuring blood pressure

↓

Symptom relief, stable blood pressure, standing slowly, observing in situ

↓

Accompanied by colleagues, enter the "take–off zone1"

↓

Follow the process to complete the procedure of removing protective equipment

↓

Leave the "take–off zone2" and give relevant symptomatic treatment

Figure 3.19   Syncope emergency treatment process in the isolation area

20. The Management Process of Sharp Instrument Injury Emergency

Quickly go to the buffer room and take off your gloves

Squeezes blood from the proximal to the distal end to the hand sink

Rinse under running water

Iodine or 75% alcohol wipe disinfection

Bandaging as appropriate for wound size

Replace with new cleaning gloves

Follow the process to complete the remove protection supplies process

Enter the clean area, disinfect again (iodine or 75% alcohol), and bandage the wound.

Report infection controllers and department directors in a timely manner, scan QR codes to report occupational exposures

Provide preventive medication according to the condition of exposure

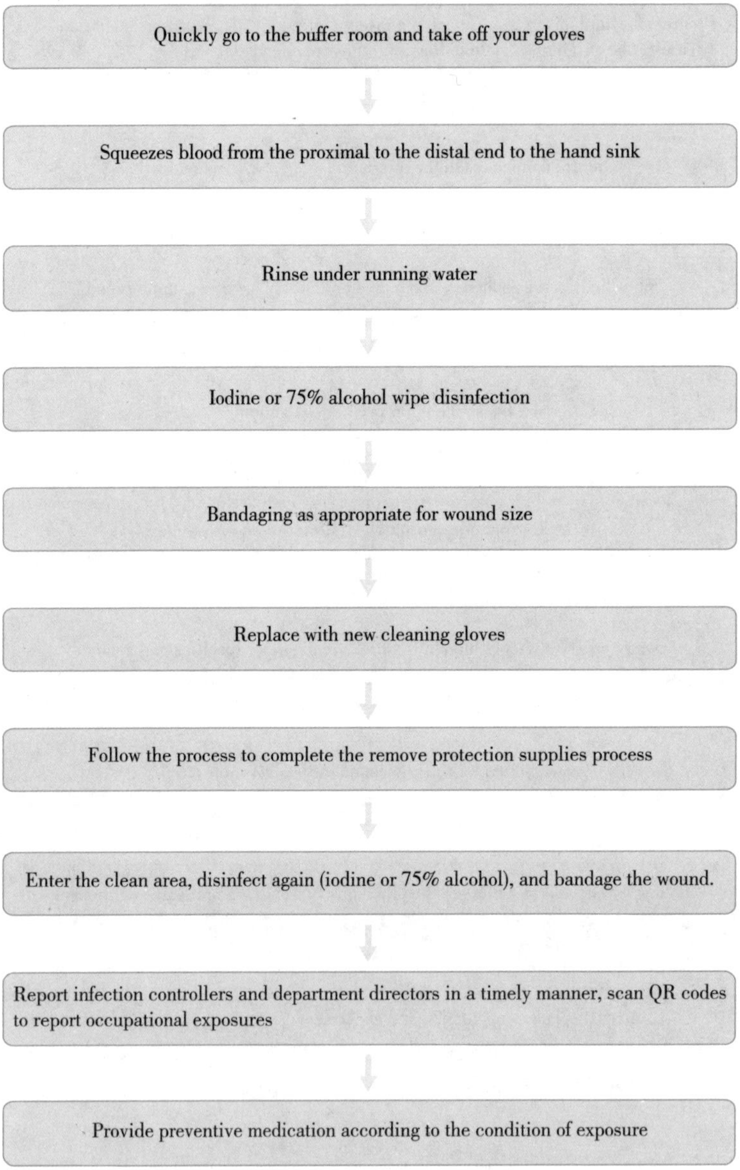

Figure 3.20   Sharp instrument injury emergency management process

21. Emergency Treatment Process for Double-layer Glove Breakage

Immediately back to "Take-off zone 1", hand hygiene

↓

Take off your two pairs of gloves

↓

Hand hygiene

↓

Re-wear clean gloves, hand hygiene

↓

Follow the instruction to complete deprotection equipment process

↓

Re-wear protective equipment to work in quarantine area

↓

Report to infection control staff and department director in time, scan QR code to report occupational exposure

Figure 3.21　Emergency treatment procedure for double-layer glove breakage

22. Occupational Exposure Treatment Process for Medical Personnel

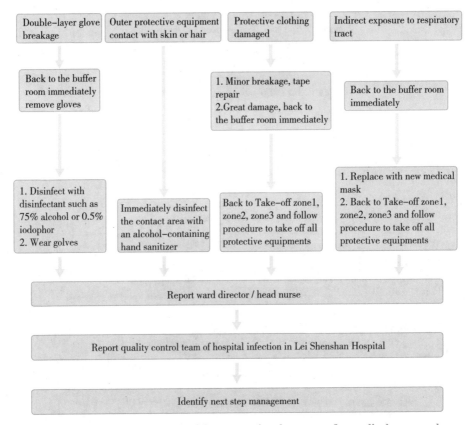

Figure 3.22   Treatment protocol for occupational exposure for medical personnel

23. The Process of Occupational Exposure Disposal for Medical Personnel

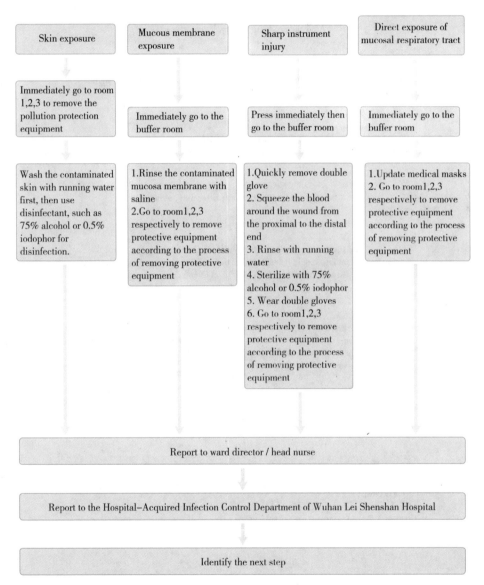

Figure 3.23   **Disposal procedure for occupational exposure for high-risk medical personnel**

24. Cleaning and Disinfection Process of Power Air Supply Device

After the power air supply device is used

↓

Hand hygiene, wipe the hood and the outside of the breathing tube with high-level disinfection wipes

↓

Hand hygiene, take off the hood gently

↓

Separate main engine, belt, filter and solenoid

↓

The hood and filter are used once. After replacing the clean sterile gloves, the following operations should be carried out: the main machine and the belt should be wiped and disinfected with high level disinfecting wipes (disinfected twice). The first cleaning, the second disinfection

↓

Replace the sterile gloves, sterilize the interface between the solenoid and the main machine host with high-level disinfection wipes ,wrap the interface with sterile gloves and seal with adhesive tape

↓

After soaking and sterilizing the solenoid, deliver it to the disinfection supply center

↓

After disinfection, the main machine and belt are sealed with clean plastic bags respectively, then placed in the clean organized box, and the battery is charged for backup

Figure 3.24   Cleaning and disinfection process of power air supply devices

25. Wuhan Leishenshan Nosocomial Infection Outbreak Reporting and Emergency Treatment Processes

Prospective monitoring of full-time staff
Clinical medical staff monitoring
Microbiology staff monitoring

3 or more cases of nosocomial infection with the same syndrome, the same source of infection and the same exposure factors

Report to the Hospital-Acquired Infection Control Department immediately byphone during working hours
Report to the total duty on duty and holidays

The Hospital-Acquired Infection Control Department arrive at the scene to investigate and verify

Confirm the outbreak

Report to hospital leadership and hospital infection management committee within one hour

The hospital infection management team and other relevant departments work closely together to actively investigate, analyze, and control

Hospital infection management committee launches plan

1. Conduct epidemiological investigations to speculate possible sources of infection, routes of transmission and factors of infection
2. Conduct etiological testing of infected cases, microbiological testing of possible sources and routes of transmission
3. Develop control measures to initially isolate the infected, the suspected infected and related contacts
4. Analyze survey data, formulate and implement targeted disinfection, isolation, and treatment measures as soon as possible

Outbreaks of more than 3 cases or more than 5 suspected cases should be reported within 12 hours
Outbreaks of more than 5 cases or cases resulting in death or personal injury should be reported within 2 hours
Outbreaks of more than 10 nosocomial infection cases, nosocomial infection with a particular or new pathogen and nosocomial infection that can have major public impact or serious consequences should be reported within 2 hours

The infection is under control and terminate the plan
Write the investigation report, formulate the next step of prevention and control, and treatment measures

Report to Jiangxia District Health Administration and CDC

Work closely with the health administration to conduct investigations and control work: including survey sampling, on-site inquiry, patient isolation, logistic support, etc.

Summarize experience and lessons and give results feedback

Figure 3.25   Outbreak reporting and emergency treatment procedures for Wuhan Leishenshan nosocomial infection

(Xiao-ping Zhu   Yi-ping Mao   Ying Wang   Ting Wang   Yong-ning Liu

Ying Xie   Gui-lan Zhai   Yan Fu   Gen-di Lu   Xiao-fang Fu   Yi-le Huang

Min Li   Hong-ying Zhang   Qian Zhong   Yong-juan Zhao)

Chapter 4 Guiding Principles for Infection Prevention and Control of Different Personnel

Part 1 Guiding Principles for Infection Prevention and Control of Medical Care Personnel

1.General Requirements for Medical Care Personnel

There are numerous medical teams in the Leishenshan Hospital, and the medical care personnel work in shifts based on the prevailing situation. Therefore, the medical care personnel on duty in the ward are required to provide the health examination results for nearly one week and are only be issued work permits and hold relevant certificates after passing the nosocomial infection training and examination.

2. Guiding Principles for the Infection and Control of the Medical Care Personnel (Enforcement Principles)

2.1 Master the layout and process of infection prevention and control in the hospital areas and wards.

2.2 Master the process of wearing and removing protective equipment and matters requiring attention.

2.3 Familiar with the daily infection prevention and control work in the ward, and earnestly implement the relevant system as per the requirements of the infection prevention and control group.

2.4 Master the relevant rules, regulations, and procedures of nosocomial infection management formulated by the hospital.

2.5 Strictly abide by the *Resident Medical Team Management System*, to ensure that the medical team living area behavior conforms to the principle of infection prevention and control.

Part 2　Guiding Principles for the Infection and Control of the Administrative Personnel

1.General Requirements for Hospital Administrative Personnel

The administrative personnel in the hospital area should provide health certificates and receive training on infection prevention and control knowledge before accessing the hospital area, and the relevant departments should issue work certificates and hold relevant certificates before taking up their posts.

The administrative personnel in the hospital area should follow the military route–administrative area according to the management of the staff and the commuting distance. If the administrative personnel need to visit the isolation ward due to their work, they should observe the entrance of the ward–medical care street–administrative area to conduct the corresponding task. Before entering the isolation ward, the administrative personnel should be familiar with the layout and process of infection prevention and control in the hospital, the layout and process of infection prevention and control in the ward, comply with the requirements of infection prevention and control in the ward, and control their behavior according to the ward management regulations.

2. Guiding Principles for Infection Prevention and Control of the Administrative Personnel (Enforcement Principles)

2.1 Master the hospital area as well as ward infection prevention and control layout and process.

2.2 Master the process of wearing and removing protective equipment and matters requiring attention.

2.3 Master the relevant rules, regulations, and procedures of nosocomial infection management formulated by the hospital.

Part 3   Guiding Principles for Infection Prevention and Control of the Cleaning Personnel

1. General Requirements for the Cleaning Personnel

Cleaning personnel in the hospital area should manage the commuting distance according to the requirements of the staff and follow the military route–the entrance of the ward–medical care street–each ward in performing the corresponding work. Cleaning personnel should be familiar with the layout and process of infection prevention and control in the hospital area, and the layout and process of infection prevention and control in the ward area. The movement lines of the cleaning personnel in the hospital area and ward area should proceed; clean–potential pollution–polluted area; Pollution area–potential pollution–clean area. It is forbidden to move at will in all the areas.

All cleaning personnel should be trained in basic knowledge of health examination and infection prevention and control and be issued with certificates before taking up their posts. The training contents include cleaning and disinfection methods and procedures, medical waste classification and collection system, occupational exposure emergency disposal procedures, hand hygiene, and proper use of personal protective equipment, etc.

2. Requirements for Cleaning and Disinfection of the Hospital Environment Floor and Object Surface

Disinfection of the hospital environment ground and surface of object should be performed according to the different zones. Sanitary ware should be used separately. Special mops should be set up in the cleaning area, contaminated area, and toilet, respectively. The mops should be clearly labeled and separately cleaned. After use, the mops should be disinfected and hung to dry to remain on standby.

2.1 Disinfection measures for clean areas

The ground and object surface in the cleaning area should be disinfected, and wet cleaning should be adopted when there is no evident contamination. When there is evident contamination, the surface should be sprayed with chlorine–containing 500 mg/L disinfectant, the visible contaminants are removed using hygroscopic materials, and then cleaned and disinfected. One towel should be used per room/area in the disinfection.

It is recommended that the disinfection be conducted not less than twice a day (including public toilets).

2.2 Disinfection measures in potentially contaminated areas

Potentially contaminated areas mainly include PPE rooms in the ward and buffer rooms leading to the ward. It is recommended to use disposable sterilized wet tissue meeting the concentration requirements of the potentially contaminated areas, one per room, and one for disposal. It is recommended to use 500 ~ 1000 mg/L chlorine–containing disinfectant to soak the dry towel for wet disinfection, at least twice a day.

2.3 Contaminated areas

Contaminated areas mainly constitute isolation wards, outer walkways, specimen storage rooms, etc. It is recommended to use 1000mg/L chlorine–containing disinfectant for wet disinfection of the ground and the surface of objects in the contaminated areas, and make one bed and one towel at least twice a day.

Whenever there is a small amount of contaminant of either blood, secretions and/or vomitus of the patient in the contaminated area, disposable absorbent materials (such as gauze, rag, etc.) are used by first dipping in chlorine–containing disinfectant solution (or disinfection wet towel or dry towel capable of achieving high–level disinfection) with chlorine (5000~10,000 mg/L) and wiping the surface. For large amounts of contamination, they should be completely covered with the disinfectant powder, or bleaching powder containing water–absorbing components, or completely covered with disposable water–absorbing materials. Then sufficient 5000~10,000mg/L chlorine–containing disinfectant solution should be poured on the water–absorbing materials for more than 30 minutes (or disinfection dry towel capable of achieving high–level disinfection), and then carefully remove.

The cleaning personnel should avoid contact with contaminants during the cleaning process, and the cleaned contaminants must be disposed of as medical waste. Secretions and vomitus of patients should be collected in special containers, soaked, and disinfected using chlorine–containing disinfectant with available chlorine of 20,000 mg/L for 2 hours according to the ratio of the substance to medicine (1:2). After removing the contaminants, disinfect the surface of the contaminated environmental objects. Containers containing contaminants should be soaked and disinfected using the chlorine–containing disinfectant solution with available chlorine of 5000mg/L for 30 minutes, and then cleaned.

3. Medical Waste Disposal Requirements

3.1 The medical waste in the isolation ward should be transported out of the isolation zone through a special channel and should be pre–disinfected or packaged again in the buffer zone before being transferred.

3.2 The delivery tools of waste disposal should be cleaned using 1000mg/L chlorine–containing disinfectant after the delivery, every day.

3.3 Whenever the delivery tools are contaminated, they should be disinfected using chlorine–containing 2000mg/L disinfectant on time. The medical waste should be sealed for temporary storage and transportation. Stacking of medical waste is strictly prohibited to prevent spillage and leakage.

3.4 The temporary storage room for medical waste should be pre–disinfected using effective chlorine content of not less than 1000mg/L disinfectant, and the ultraviolet light irradiation increased for not less than 1 hour.

3.5 When handling medical waste, the transport and cleaning personnel must wear protective clothing, gloves, masks, boots, and other protective equipment. After the disposal work is completed, the equipment and protective equipment must be disinfected.

4. Requirements for Handling Emergencies

4.1 In the case of leakage of medical waste, the contaminated site ground should be sprayed with 2000mg/L chlorine–containing disinfectant, cleaned, and disinfected. The disinfection should be performed, starting from the least contaminated area to the most contaminated area. All used tools that may be contaminated should be disinfected.

4.2 If any of the medical waste transporters gets accidentally injured in the process of disposing medical waste, emergency treatment should be carried based on the process of occupational exposure.

4.3 In case a patient carelessly walks out of the isolation area, all places and appliances in close contact with the patient should be disinfected using a disinfectant with available chlorine content of not less than 2000mg/L.

4.4 In case of a fire outbreak in the isolation zone, and after the fire is controlled, the post–disaster site and all places and appliances in close contact with the evacuated patients should be disinfected using a disinfectant with available chlorine content of not less than 2000mg/L.

5. Principles of Life Management for Cleaning Personnel

Cleaning personnel working in the hospital area should strengthen their self–management awareness, and their accommodation should be kept clean and tidy, ventilated frequently, and disinfected regularly. In the case of contamination, the room should be cleaned and disinfected immediately. Cleaning personnel should gathering in large numbers in one room. If personnel have physical discomfort symptoms, they should report as per the *Health Management System.*

Part 4　Guiding Principles for Infection Prevention and Control of the Security Personnel

1. General Requirements for the Hospital Security Personnel

The security personnel in the hospital area should provide health certificates and receive training on infection prevention and control knowledge before accessing the hospital area, and the relevant departments should issue work certificates after assessment. The security personnel of the hospital should hold applicable certificates.

The security personnel in the hospital area should manage their commuting distance according to the requirements of the staff, and proceed through the military route–the entrance of the ward–medical care street–each ward in performing their work. The security personnel should be familiar with the layout and process of infection prevention and control in the hospital area as well as the layout and process of infection prevention and control in the ward area. Under normal circumstances, security personnel should work at the entrance of the clean area and the main entrances and exits of the Leishenshan Hospital. In case the security personnel is required to enter the ward, their movement route should proceed through; the clean area –potentially contaminated– contaminated area; contaminated area–potentially contaminated–clean area. All the security personnel are forbidden from moving at will in all areas.

2.Guiding Principles for Infection Prevention and Control of Security Personnel (Enforcement Principles)

2.1 Master the hospital area and ward infection prevention and control layout and process.

2.2 Master the process of wearing and removing protective equipment and matters requiring attention.

2.3 Strictly adhere to the work responsibilities; strictly and thoroughly screen the temperature of all medical personnel and administrative personnel at the entrances in the hospital.

2.4 Strictly adhere to the work responsibilities; strictly inspect the certificates of different staff in the hospital area.

2.5 Master the core nosocomial infection prevention and control systems and processes, including occupational exposure emergency treatment process, hand hygiene, correct use of personal protective equipment, etc.

Part 5   Guiding Principles for Infection Prevention and Control of Maintenance Personnel

1.General Requirements for Hospital Maintenance Personnel

Maintenance personnel in the hospital area should provide health certificates when accessing the hospital area. The maintenance personnel must pass the training and assessment on infection prevention and control knowledge. The relevant departments should issue work certificates to the maintenance personnel before assigning them tasks. The maintenance personnel should hold relevant certificates before taking up their posts.

Maintenance personnel in the hospital area should manage their commuting distance according to the staff requirements. The maintenance personnel should proceed through the military road–the entrance of the ward–medical care street– each ward in performing their duties. Maintenance personnel should be familiar with the layout and process of infection prevention and control in the hospital area, and the layout and process of infection prevention and control in the ward area. The movement route of maintenance personnel in the hospital area and wards entails; clean–potentially contaminated–contaminated area; contaminated area–potentially contaminated–clean area. All maintenance personnel are forbidden from moving at will in all the areas.

2.Guiding Principles for Infection Prevention and Control of
Maintenance Personnel (Enforcement Principle)

2.1 Master the hospital area and ward infection prevention and control layout
and process.

2.2 Master the process of wearing and removing protective equipment and
matters needing attention.

2.3 It is recommended to keep a set of commonly used maintenance equipment
in the instrument room of each ward. When the equipment must be taken out, it must
be soaked or wiped with 1000mg/L chlorine-containing disinfectant and should be
taken out only after 30 minutes.

2.4 Master the core nosocomial infection prevention and control systems and
processes, including occupational exposure emergency treatment process, hand
hygiene, and correct use of personal protective equipment.

Part 6   Guiding Principles for Infection Prevention and Control of Temporary Personnel

1.General Requirements for Hospital Temporary Personnel

Temporary personnel in the hospital area include but are not limited to personnel
who visit the hospital temporarily on business, journalists, volunteers, etc. Temporary
personnel entering the hospital area should be registered and put on temporary work
permits. The temporary personnel in the hospital area should strictly comply with
the requirements of infection prevention and control and wear different levels of
protective equipment as per the respective movement route.

2.Guiding Principles for Infection Prevention and Control of
Temporary Personnel (Enforcement Principle)

2.1 Under the guidance of the hospital staff, temporary personnel should familiarize themselves with the hospital and ward infection prevention and control layout and process.

2.2 Under the guidance of the ward infection prevention and control supervisor, temporary personnel, should correctly wear and remove protective equipment and matters requiring attention to be correctly conducted.

2.3 A record of the materials, instruments, and equipment to be delivered into the ward should be provided to the QC infection prevention and control group in advance, and the disinfection standard of the ward must be strictly observed.

2.4 Instruments and equipment to be taken out of the ward should be soaked or wiped with 1000mg/L chlorine-containing disinfectant before, or wiped with 75% alcohol and left for 30 minutes before taking them out.

(Ying Wang   Fei Gong)

Chapter 5   Working Mode

Part 1   Spots-setting Quality Control in Wards

Spots-setting work mode is classifying the wards into different infection risks areas. This helps to determine the contents of supervision based on the requirements of sensory control in each area.

1. Wards are categorized into 3 areas based on their risk level: low-risk area (clean area), medium-risk area (potential polluted area) and high-risk area (polluted area).

2. The low-risk area is the rest room for medical staff. Infection control inspector conducts hand hygiene execution and environmental disinfection checks at least once a day.

3. Medium-risk areas are doctors and nurses' offices, bathing and changing areas. Infection control monitors carry out inspections of hand hygiene execution, the use of protective equipment for medical personnel, disposal of fabrics after use, slippers and environmental disinfection at least twice a day.

4. The high-risk areas are the isolation wards; the first and second off zones. Infection control monitors conduct inspections of enforcement of hand hygiene execution, protective equipment use and removal procedures, medical waste disposal and environmental disinfection at least twice a day.

5. The problems encountered are recorded timely. Feedback and rectification measures are then put in place and the rectification effect evaluated.

Part 2　"Problem-oriented" Working Mode

1. Introduction to Problem Orientated Working Mode

Problem orientation originates from curriculum design and teaching work. It is a teaching form in which the knowledge learned is applied to solve practical problems under the guidance of teachers and on the premise of independent learning and cooperative discussion of students. Currently, problem-oriented thinking has been widely used in all kinds of work. It is a daily use, efficient and easy-to-operate working mode.

The success of the problem-oriented mode of work depends on consciously establishing the problem, fundamentally focusing on solving the problem, proper tracing of the problem source, understanding the cause and effect of the problem, finding the true nature of the problem, and exploring the path and strategy to solve the problem. Its operation mechanism follows the path of: finding problems, analyzing problems, solving problems and evaluating the effects of the solution.

2. Application of "Problem orientation" Working Mode in Controlling Nosocomial Infections at Leishenshan Hospital

At Leishenshan Hospital, there are many medical teams facing complicated problems. Continuing with operations in the conventional way could lead to numerous challenges during an epidemic control. This necessitates the adjustment of the working mode. Problem-oriented working mode can lessen the burden of such infections control works as well as encourage a more homogenic management of the team.

2.1 Finding the problem

This is the first step of the problem-oriented working mode. In this step, focus should be put on all members of the hospital including medical staff, administrative staff, logistic support staff and patients. Leishenshan Hospital is faced with varying infection control problems from time to time. As such, it needs to be good at finding the problems. The nosocomial infection management team should summarize the outstanding issues identified by each department in a timely manner and focus on how to classify and deal with them. The issue can be classified as either an environmental layout issue, a process issue or a security issue among others.

2.2 Analysis of the problem

The nosocomial infection management team classifies the severity of the outstanding problems identified at this stage. The team should analyze the problems found, the urgency of the problems, the severity of the problems, and the departments that need to work together to solve the problems. It then submits the urgent and serious problems to the Nosocomial Infection Management Committee for discussion. The Nosocomial Infection Management Committee discusses the solutions to the problems submitted and outlines the merits and demerits of various solutions. Appropriate solutions to the problems are then finally formulated by the committee.

2.3 Solving the problems

The nosocomial infection management team holds a problem orientation work coordination meeting on the solutions formulated by the Nosocomial Infection Management Committee. Based on the nature of the problem to be solved, multiple departments such as the comprehensive coordination group, medical service group, nursing group, logistics support group, and security group are invited to the meeting. The team communicates the solutions formulated by the Nosocomial Infection Management Committee to the other attendees and propose technical solutions and time limits for solving the problems. The coordination meeting can be held multiple times in the process of problem solving based on the magnitude of the problem. The meetings are geared to assess the progress made in problem solving, problems found, and the problems that require coordination and resolution of other departments until the problems are resolved. Quality management tools such as PDCA, Gantt chart and QCC are commonly used to solve problems in the "problem-oriented" working mode.

2.4 Evaluation of the effects of the solution

After the problem is solved, the nosocomial infection management team reports the solution process and its effect to the Nosocomial Infection Management Committee. The committee evaluates the effects of the solutions through expert discussion and put forward the key points and ideas for the next work.

3. Case Sharing

During the early stages of construction of Leishenshan Hospital, disinfection was not fully implemented. This problem was identified by the nosocomial infection management team which carried out an in-depth research to prevent healthcare-acquired infections. Disinfection measures were implemented to solve the problem based on the "problem-oriented work mode.

3.1 Discovering the problem

The main cause of inadequate disinfection measures was insufficient training of cleaning staff. This had been caused by inadequate pre-job training for new cleaners, low awareness of hand hygiene, unfamiliar use of personal protective equipment, lack of proper cleaning procedures and methods and irregular use of cleaning instruments among other causes.

3.2 Analysis of the problem

After identification and clarification of the problem, the nosocomial infection management team reported their findings to the Nosocomial Infection Management Committee. Several measures to solve the problem were presented in the report. There was a need for systematic training of cleaners on hand hygiene, use of protective equipment, hospital district, ward district, disinfectant configuration and cleaning process. There was also a need for process development in regard to cleaner responsibilities, cleaners induction training system, SOP of cleaning and cleaning quality supervision form among others. Further to this, continuous intensive training, continuous strengthening training using visualized " cleaning workflows" and

" cleaning tool classification requirements" publicity maps, daily supervision and quality control were needed. The inspection content included mastery of new sensory control knowledge related to COVID-19, steps and procedures for cleaning different areas, the correctness of wearing and removing personal protective equipment, use and configuration of disinfectant and disposal of cleaning supplies among others. The relevant content was reflected in the "cleaning quality inspection form" .

3.3 Solving the problem

Based on the solutions formulated by the Nosocomial Infection Management Committee to prevent healthcare-acquired infections, the nosocomial infection management team held a coordination group meeting to divide the work amongst the relevant departments for effective problem solving. The departments included the medical team, the nursing team, the logistics support team, the person in charge of the cleaning company and the ward quality sense controller. Supervision of all departments was conducted simultaneously during the problem solving process. The quality control and the collaborative departments discussed and analyzed the reasons of occurrence of problems detected during inspection. They further formulated the improvement plan again and put the improved method into use again to observe the effect. This form of quality improvement was continuous to ensure healthy operation of the PDCA cycle.

3.4 Evaluation of effectiveness of the solutions

Various inspection indicators such as hand hygiene performance, wear and tear accuracy of protective equipment, disinfectant preparation, and cleaning and disinfection pass rate were compared with the previous ones to gauge improvement. Statistical methods were used were necessary to understand the effects of continuous improvement.

Part 3   Informatization Monitoring System

Medical infection prevention and control management information system aims to effectively prevent and control infection, improve medical quality, and ensure medical safety. It is based on the norms, standards and guidelines for nosocomial infection prevention and control. It monitors infection-related factors for hospital-wide patients by retrieving suspected infection cases, providing early warning information on infection outbreaks, establishing an infection report management platform, collecting and analyzing the occurrence of infection statistically, establishing a targeted monitoring platform to monitor the process of vulnerable patients, improving infection protection measures and reducing the infection rate.

One of the infection prevention and control modes of Leishenshan Hospital is the comprehensive realization of information-based surveillance. It includes the following aspects:

1. Comprehensive Monitoring

Based on infection diagnostic standards, data standardization and empirical values, accurate screening of relevant infection indicators for hospitalized patients should be done. The infection management department manages the hospital's suspected infection indicators and suspected infected patients. The department is also tasked with treatment and protection of infected patients.

2. Targeted Monitoring

This focuses on monitoring highly infectious and vulnerable populations. It also offers special monitoring of the ICU, key surgery theatres and multi-drug-resistant bacteria. It guides the protection of patients from infections based on the analysis of infection indicators.

3. Environmental Hygiene Monitoring

Environmental hygiene monitoring implements the full process of infection management. It encompasses application of the corrective measures, monitoring their impact, giving a result feedback and statistical analysis of the effectiveness of the corrective measures. This facilitates clinical self-examination and targeted work of the infection management department.

4. Hand Hygiene Monitoring

This focuses on the implementation of hand hygiene compliance surveys, hand hygiene product maintenance, hand hygiene product consumption registration, hand hygiene consumption statistics, hand hygiene compliance rate and other query statistics. There should be high accuracy and consistency of these data. Hand hygiene indicators of wearing and removing personal protective equipment have been included at Leishenshan Hospital.

5. Occupational Exposure Monitoring

The clinical department reports any occupational exposures to facilitate follow-up and treatment. This is based on the occupational exposure process.

6. Protective Equipment Monitoring

This is the characteristic monitoring index of Leishenshan Hospital. Health workers are required to wear and remove personal protective equipment 100% correctly. The process is guided using a real time electronic video in which a staff can obtain the guidance of the full operation process. Moreover, an effective and convenient mobile cloud monitoring service is added to this system to facilitate proper wearing and removal of PPE's when the staff is not in the cleaning area.

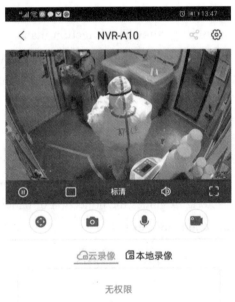

Figure 5.1　Real-time image of cloud monitoring of wearing and removal of personal protective equipment

(Ying Wang Peng Wang Bi-long Feng Kun Li)

Chapter 6　Management of Resident Medical Team

Part 1　Establishment of an Infection Control Group

Immediately after the establishment of a medical team for aid in Hubei province, an infection control group comprising of a full-time infection control staff or an infection control nurse should be set up. The infection control group under the leadership of a medical team captain is responsible for infection prevention and control training of the medical team members as well as infection control work at the hospital and resident station.

The infection control team immediately investigates the resident station and hospital immediately after arrival to formulate the resident station's infection prevention and control measures based on the actual situation. The team then submit the findings to the leading group of the medical team for review and release. The team is also responsible for regular supervision and random inspections to ensure proper implementation of the prevention and control measures.

Part 2　Resident Station Lodging Protocol

1. Leaving the Lodging for Work

1.1 Wear inner clothing (no special requirements, keep warm and comfortable).

1.2 Change outer clothing and shoes, and wear a surgical mask (also carry a surgical mask).

1.3 Use an alcohol-based quick-drying disinfectant near the elevator for hand sanitation when leaving the lodging or entering the hospital using an elevator (or touch the elevator button using a paper towel).

1.4 After arriving at the hospital, take off your outer clothing and shoes in the locker room of the clean zone for medical staff and wear the appropriate work clothes and shoes. Take off the work cloths when entering a potentially contaminated area and wear personal protective equipment correctly.

2. Going Back to the Lodging

2.1 Takeoff personal protective equipment following the correct procedure and wear a new surgical mask. Put on outwear and shoes and follow proper hand hygiene measures before leaving the hospital. Pay attention to hand hygiene after touching elevator buttons or other public utilities.

2.2 Use alcohol-based quick-drying hand disinfectant for hand hygiene on arrival at the lodging entrance. Remove the mask worn at the hospital and discard it into the dedicated trash bin deployed at the entrance of the lodging.

2.3 Sanitize your hands and wear a new surgical mask.

2.4 Get your body temperature taken using a body thermometer gun provided at the entrance for testing each other's temperature. Any temperature abnormality should be reported to the infection control committee immediately. Sanitize your hands after the temperature test and proceed to your room.

2.5 Use an alcohol-based quick-drying disinfectant near the elevator for hand sanitation before entering your room if using an elevator (or touch the elevator button using a paper towel).

3. Entering the Lodging Room

3.1 The room is divided and classified into several areas. The entrance is a non-clean section (note that it is not a hospital's contaminated area to avoid confusion). The bathroom is a cleaning area. The interior of the room is a clean-living area (including beds, sofas, tables and chairs).

3.2 Take off your outer clothing after entering your room and hang it on a lateral of the closet immediately (split the room of closet in half, this lateral is a non–clean area). Take off your shoes and put them in the bottom grid of the closet. Put on your slippers and take off your pants. If there is no closet, you can put it in a cardboard box or basket and then put it in the corner behind the door. You can also hang out clothes outside the door (if there is a hook or coat rack) and put shoes outside the door.

3.3 When entering the bathroom (washing area), wash your hands before taking a bath. Pay attention to cleaning the ear canal, nasal cavity and eyes. Using alcohol-based or iodophor disinfectants is not recommended because they may damage the skin and mucosal microbiota. They can cause mucosal irritation thus leading to mucosal damage which may increase the risk of pathogen invasion. In case of suspicious contamination or exposure after returning to the lodging, emergency treatment at the hospital is not adequate to minimize exposure. Instead, the skin can be cleansed and disinfected using chemical disinfectants such as 0.5% iodophor, alcohol–based disinfectants and hydrogen peroxide. The mucous membrane can be rinsed with 0.05% iodophor or normal saline. Spectacle wearers also need to disinfect the spectacles. If the cleaning area of the local hospital has a bathroom and it is far from the lodging, you can take a bath at the hospital cleaning area and return to work. It is however recommended to shower in the lodging room to avoid sharing the bathroom if the lodging is closer to hospital. This is highly recommended if the lodging has no suspicious contamination or infection.

3.4 Put on clean clothes and shoes before entering the clean–living area.

3.5 Outerwear can be washed and dried using a washing machine provided by the lodging (washing liquid containing disinfection can be used). The inner clothes are washed in the bathroom by self. If there is suspected contamination, it is recommended that you discard the clothes. If you have to reuse them, soak and disinfect the clothes with a disinfectant containing between 250 and 500mg/L of chlorine for 30 minutes and then rinse them with clean water.

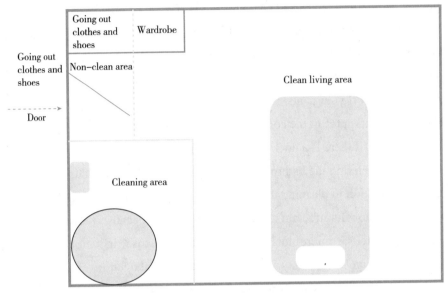

Figure 6.1   Room partition diagram of the assistant medical team members

4. Eating

4.1 Avoid gathering and eating together at the lodging's restaurant. Carry food back to your room.

4.2 Surgical masks (no need to wear N95 masks) must be worn and quick-drying hand disinfectants used in the restaurant entrance before and after taking food to ensure proper hand hygiene.

4.3 Avoid going out of the lodging compound to take food. Clean clothes should be worn when going to take food.

4.4 If you are eating in a lodging restaurant, choose to eat at different periods when there are fewer people. Avoid eating opposite each other as well as talking. Sit more than 1.5 meters apart. Fold the removed mask from inside and wrap it with paper towels as you eat to prevent contamination.

4.5 Avoid eating at the hospital. If you have to do so, eat when there are fewer people, keep an adequate distance and avoid talking. Eat from the designated areas.

Part 3   Management of Personnel Behavior

1. Avoid meeting with relatives and friends for personal reasons. Contact them by telephone, wechat and other network channels.

2. Avoid going out for personal reasons and going out alone. Report to the team leader if it's very necessary to go out.

3. Masks must be worn at all time when leaving the room (including inside the hotel compound and meeting rooms).

4. Minimize the number of physical meetings. Instead, hold virtual meetings. Put an end to recreational parties and avoid visiting colleagues. Keep a distance and avoid shaking hands when having face-to-face conversations.

5. Smokers should minimize smoking. Smoke at the designated areas. 2 or more people should avoid smoking at the same time.

6. Team members should monitor their body temperature and physical symptoms daily. Any abnormality should be reported immediately to the infection control team.

7. Garbage in the rooms should be timely dumped in the garbage can deployed in the stairwell of each floor.

8. Keep warm and ensure good sleep and rest. Take adequate amounts of water, and eat more fruits and vegetables.

9. Each team member should be accommodated individually to reduce the risk of cross infection.

Part 4   Cleaning and Disinfection

1.Air Purification and Disinfection

There's no need to purify air without airborne contaminants. Ensure there is adequate indoor air circulation by leaving the doors and windows open for 30 minutes twice or thrice a day. Don't use a central air-conditioning system in the resident station unless under the guidance of professional managers. Independent air-conditioning systems can be used.

2.Floor Cleaning and Disinfection

Elevators, corridors and room floors should be sprayed with disinfectant by the local personnel. Chlorine dioxide or chlorine-containing disinfectants are recommended. Chlorine concentration should be between 250 and 500mg/L. If there's no unified disinfection, clean and disinfect your room or working area using the indicated disinfectant on your own. Open the doors and windows to allow air circulation. This reduces irritation after disinfection. Wash off the disinfectant using clean water after taking effect for 30 minutes.

3. Cleaning and Disinfection of Object Surfaces

Wipe indoor object surfaces with disinfectant wipes or 75% alcohol. The key areas refer to the high-frequency contacting surfaces such as bathroom doorknobs, light switches, tables, mobile phones and room cards (Chlorinated disinfectants are not recommended to wiping because their causticity is strong and acting time is long). Keep away from naked fire flames when using alcohol for safety.

4.Cloth Washing and Disinfection

Clothes should be washed frequently. It's not recommended to spray clothing and shoes, because the disinfectant can damage respiratory mucosa. Moreover, there is no evidence-based medical proofs show that clothes and shoes are important vectors of the virus. Cognizant to this, the most important step is to clean and disinfect the hands that touch the clothes and shoes.

5.Hand Hygiene

It is necessary to provide alcohol-based hand disinfectants in the rooms and the station's public areas such as near the doorways, at the elevator landing, in elevator-lift rooms and restaurant. Team members should clean their hands after touching public surfaces.

6.Vehicle Cleaning and Disinfection

The team's station and hospital should be close to each other and have a dedicated transport vehicle. The infection control team should ensure daily cleaning and disinfection of the vehicle to keep all the inner surfaces clean. A disinfectant containing 500mg/L of chlorine is recommended for wiping and disinfecting the vehicle once a day. Clean water should be used to wash off the disinfectant after 30 minutes of action.

Part 5   Monitoring Infections and Emergency Procedures

1.Self-monitoring of Temperature and Physical Symptoms

Each team member should self-monitor their body temperature daily. Fever is considered if body temperature is above 37.3 ℃ . Team members should also monitor other typical symptoms such as dry cough, chest tightness, dyspnea, fatigue and diarrhea (excluding diet and stress factors). A team member should immediately report to the infection prevention and control group if they have any of such symptoms.

2.Daily Health Questionnaire

The infection prevention and control group should develop a daily health questionnaire for the medical team. Each member of the medical team should fill it out consciously and truthfully every day.

3.Daily Health Assessment

The medical team should set up an infection assessment expert group consisting of respiratory, infectious and critical medical experts. The infection prevention and control group should collect the health questionnaires of the team members daily, give a list of symptomatic team members to the infection assessment expert group, and inform the symptomatic team members to return to their rooms immediately for isolation. The isolated members must rest in a confined place and avoid going out. Meals can be delivered using plastic bags and hanged on the door handle outside the door for the isolated members to pick. The isolated members should then be evaluated individually by the expert group.

4.Assessment of the Risk Factors and Symptoms

Risk assessment is based on risk factors and symptoms.

① Risk factors are hazardous exposures when at work such as masks falling off, damage of protective clothing, exposure of the mucous membrane, sharp injuries and close contact with infected persons without protection among others.

② Typical symptoms include fever, dry cough, chest tightness, dyspnea, fatigue and diarrhea (excluding diet and stress factors).

③ Other symptoms include runny nose, sneezing and sore throat (especially accompanied by cold history).

Members who have undergone ① and those exhibiting ② are at a high risk of having been infected. Chest CT examination must be performed. If CT imaging shows high suspicion of infection, nucleic acid test must be performed immediately. Close observation is recommended for members exhibiting ②. If any further discomfort is found, then a chest CT examination must be performed. Members exhibiting ③ are at a low risk of having been infected. Close observation, symptomatic treatment, and self-isolation is recommended for their case. The release time of the isolated members is determined by the expert group based on individual assessment and the novel coronavirus pneumonia diagnosis and treatment plan.

If the nucleic acid test shows positive results, the expert group reassesses the case and take further actions. The infection prevention and control group immediately conducts an epidemiological investigation of the confirmed team members, carry out a risk assessment on those who had contact with the confirmed team members and identify those at high risk (for example those they ate with at the same table at the same time, those they talked to closely without wearing a mask, those who they shook hands with and didn't sanitize after and those they share with unsterilized items). Individual isolation is recommended for the close contacts. Those exhibiting suspicious symptoms are immediately evaluated by the expert group for further testing.

(Shi-chao Zhu)

Appendix

Appendix 1   Guidelines for Infection Control and Surveillance in Wuhan Leishenshan Hospital (First Edition)

Wuhan Leishenshan Hospital is the designated hospital for the treatment of COVID-19. This special hospital was designed in a timely manner to offer effective surveillance system for infection prevention and control of nosocomial infections. During the epidemic period, monitoring, prevention and control of nosocomial infections in Wuhan Leishenshan Hospital were implemented while conforming to the characteristics and practical conditions of an hospital. Therefore, the components of the monitoring procedures conform with the measures for the management, prevention and control of nosocomial infection. The standards for the monitoring of nosocomial infection prevention and control, WS / T312-2009, as well as the technical specifications for hospital isolation, WS / T311-2009 are integrated into the special situation of Leishenshan Hospital, and the first edition of Wuhan Leishenshan Hospital infection prevention and control monitoring content was specially formulated for each ward.

● Mandatory indicators should be implemented in all wards and signed by the ward head.

● The recommended index should be monitored according to the actual situation of the wards.

● Indicators corresponding to the special infection prevention and control monitoring at Wuhan Leishenshan Hospital are monitored on a daily basis, summarized and presented to the infection prevention and control office on a weekly basis.

● Other recommended monitoring indicators should be assessed in accordance with the standards for the monitoring of nosocomial infection prevention and control, WS / T312–2009.

● In addition to new pneumonia caused by coronavirus, an outbreak of nosocomial infection was noted.

● Five compulsory indicators of infection prevention and control monitoring should be monitored in the entire disease room.

● Recommended monitoring indicators should be selectively assessed according to the actual situation.

1.Surveillance Indicators of Compulsory Infection Prevention and Control in Wuhan Leishenshan Hospital

1.1 Qualified rate of wearing protective equipment (mandatory)

Index requirement: 100%

Calculation formula: Qualified rate of wearing protective equipment = the number of medical personnel meeting the qualified wearing rate of protective equipment in the inspection/the number of medical personnel wearing protective equipment in the inspection *100%

Monitoring operation requirements:

ⅰ. It is recommended that the infection prevention and control quality control personnel in the ward monitor the wearing condition of the protective equipment of each staff who is about to enter the isolation area every shift each day, record the total number of those wearing protective equipment, the number of wearing protective equipment correctly, and prepare statistics. If there is any difficulty of wearing PPE in the disease area, random inspection should be carried out. The number of people monitored every day should not be less than 60% of the number of people entering the isolated disease area on that day.

ⅱ. If unqualified medical personnel are found in time, guidance and correction should be given on site in time.

ⅲ. The mandatory accuracy rate is 100%.

Monitoring record form:

ⅰ. It is recommended that a register of wearing protective equipment in the office area and wearing protective equipment area be established (according to the situation of the Department).

ⅱ. Each ward should summarize and report the data to the infection prevention and control office every week.

1.2 Qualified rate of protective equipment unloading (mandatory)

Index requirement: 100%

Calculation formula: Qualified rate of protective equipment removal = the number of medical personnel meeting the qualified wearing rate of protective equipment unloading in the inspection /the number of medical personnel wearing protective equipment removing in the inspection *100%

Monitoring operation requirements:

ⅰ. It is recommended that the infection prevention and control quality control personnel in the ward monitor the removal procedures for the protective materials by each staff who is about to leave the isolation area (one unloading area) in each shift every day, record the total number of people who are about to leave the isolation area, the correct number of people who are about to remove, and prepare statistics. If there is any difficulty in the disease area, random inspection should be carried out. The number of people monitored every day should not be less than 60% of the number of people entering the isolated disease area on that day.

ⅱ. If unqualified medical personnel are found in time, on-site guidance and correction should be provided in time.

ⅲ. The mandatory accuracy rate is 100%.

Monitoring record form:

ⅰ. It is recommended to set up a register to record the removal status of protective materials in the office area of the ward (according to the situation of the Department).

ⅱ. Each ward should summarize and report the data to the infection prevention and control office every week.

1.3 Hand hygiene compliance (mandatory)

Calculation formula: Hand hygiene compliance = Number of implementation opportunities of hand hygiene/ Number of hand hygiene opportunities that should be implemented*100%

Monitoring operation requirements:

ⅰ. For each shift in a given day, the controller of the quality of infection prevention and control in the entire ward should carry out random checks for the state of hand hygiene among staff in the ward and calculate the compliance.

ⅱ. The controller should identify personnel not correctly observing hand hygiene in time, give timely guidance and correction on site.

Monitoring record form:

ⅰ. It is recommended that a hand hygiene monitoring registration form should be put in the office area of the ward (according to the situation of the Department).

ⅱ. Each ward should summarize and report the data to the infection prevention and control office every week.

1.4 Hand hygiene accuracy (mandatory)

Hand hygiene accuracy is calculated using the formula: = Timing of right–hand hygiene/ Timing of hand hygiene *100%

Requirements of monitoring operations:

ⅰ. Every day, monitor in charge of the infection prevention and control (monitoring group leader or head nurse) in the entire ward should carry out random checks for the status of hand hygiene among staff in the ward and calculate the hand hygiene rate.

ⅱ. The monitor should find out the personnel not observing hand hygiene provide timely guidance and correction on site.

Monitoring record form:

ⅰ. It is recommended that a hand hygiene monitoring registry form be established in the office area of the ward (according to the situation of the Department).

ⅱ. Each ward should summarize and report the data to the infection prevention and control office every week.

1.5 Monitoring, prevention and control of outbreaks for other medical infections except COVID-19 (mandatory).

Monitoring requirements:

ⅰ. New coronavirus pneumonia should be highly noticed in clinical practice.

ⅱ. In clinical practice, medical personnel should report to the office of infection prevention and control every day the distribution of infection cases. If there are 3 or more cases of syndrome, they should be reported to the office of infection prevention and control within 2 hours.

ⅲ. Reporting cases during off duty time to the hospital.

ⅳ. The infection prevention and control office should conduct epidemiological investigation on the suspected cases of infection, and the clinical departments should cooperate with the reporting officer.

2.Contents of Infection Control and Surveillance Recommended by Doctors in Wuhan Leishenshan Hospital

Other isolated disease areas selectively carry out hospital wide monitoring and targeted monitoring according to the conditions of patients in the disease area, and in accordance with the monitoring standards of infection prevention and control.

2.1 Content of Monitoring protocols

2.1.1 Comprehensive monitoring of the entire hospital: Investigation on the prevalence of infection.

2.1.2 Targeted monitoring.

ⅰ. Surgical site monitoring.

ⅱ. Surveillance of infection prevention and control in adult ICU.

ⅲ. Bacterial resistance monitoring.

2.2 Monitoring requirements

The monitoring content is applied in line with the information monitoring work mode. Realize information monitoring.

Appendix 2 Quality Inspection and Continuous Improvement of Infection Prevention and Control Records in Wuhan Leishenshan Hospital

Department:		Ward:
Inspection topics		
Inspection contents		
Inspection feedback	Problems or achievements	
	Improvement measures	
Signature of inspector		Signature of responsible person
Date of inspection		
Evaluate the effectiveness of continuous improvement of existing problems (departments or functional departments)		
Signature of supervisor (Department):		Signature of supervisor (functional department)
Date of supervision:		
Note: this form is made in duplicate, one for the inspection department and one for the inspected department.		

Appendix 3　Hand Hygiene Monitoring Form

Number	Date	Name	Hand hygiene indication							Result	
			Before contact patient	After touching the patient / surrounding environment	Before aseptic operation	After contact with bodily fluids	After exposure to the surrounding environment	Wearing protective equipment	Protective equipment unloading	Compliance	Accuracy

Total:　Compliance rate:　　　Accuracy rate:　　　Signature of Ward head:

Appendix 4　Inspection List of Infection Control in Leishenshan Hospital

Ward patrol form of quality and infection control in Leishenshan in Wuhan

Ward:			Time:		Inspections by:			Total:	
Project	Location	Content	Points inspections	Scoring criteria	Implement	Not implemented	Problem	Score
Hospital ward infection inspection	Health care workers Avenue	Ward exterior walkway clean	1. Walkways clean and tidy	1 point				
			2. The fire exit walkway between the outer door is closed bis	2 points				
			3. The end door closed	2 points				
		No garbage piling up	1. Loitering and no garbage piled materials	2 points				
	Lounge Material channel	Staff behavior, wearing compliant	1. No aggregation behavior	2 points				
			2. Wearing outgoing clothes (forbidden to wear protective suits and gowns before going out)	2 points				
		No garbage piling up, no extraneous items pile up	1. No extraneous items pile up	2 points				
			2. Transfer recording including wash clothing, goggles, etc.	2 points				
			3. Bilateral doors closed	2 points				

Continuous the table

Ward:		Time:		Inspections by:				Total:	
Project	Location	Content	Points inspections	Scoring criteria	Implement	Not implemented	Problem	Score
Hospital ward infection inspection	Ward clean area	Clean environment	1. The environment should be clean and items displayed orderly	2 points				
		Meet the requirements of garbage	1. Clean areas with black garbage bags, potentially contaminated and contaminated medical waste in yellow bags	2 points				
		Medical waste placed according to the requirements	1. The registration record book for medical waste	1 point				
			2. Medical waste collected in double yellow bags for transport	2 points				
			3. Temporary storage of medical waste	2 points				
			4. Temporary storage of living garbage	2 points				
		Protective equipment placed in suitable place, storage in ready	1. Protective equipment placed orderly and well identified	2 points				

Continuous the table

Project	Location	Content	Points inspections	Scoring criteria	Implement	Not implemented	Problem	Score
	Ward:	Time:		Inspections by:			Total:	
Hospital ward infection inspection	Ward clean area	Protective wear and off according to the requirements	1. Wearing procedure of the protective equipment in a proper way	2 points				
			2. Wearing procedure paste on the wall	1 point				
			3. Has the mirror	1 point				
			4. Wearing protective supplies are monitored and recorded	2 points				
		Disinfection supplies storage reasonable, in line with the required concentration	1. Disinfection supplies placing reasonable	2 points				
			2. The correct concentration of disinfectant	2 points				
			3. Disinfection frequency meet the requirements	2 points				
		Office tidy and clean	1. Tidy office	2 points				

Continuous the table

Ward:		Time:		Inspections by:				Total:	
Project	Location	Content	Points inspections	Scoring criteria	Implement	Not implemented	Problem	Score
Hospital ward infection inspection	Ward clean area	The office staff conduct compliant: Perform hand hygiene, wearing gloves if there is the use of computers, whether inadequate protection (wear protective clothing when working)	1. Never wear protective clothing at work	2 points				
			2. Do not wear gloves when using computer	2 points				
			3. Random checks for hand hygiene	2 points				
			4. Prohibiting eating in the office	2 points				
	Treatment room	Aseptic operation	1. Aseptic procedures	2 points				
			2. Randomly check hand hygiene	2 points				

Continuous the table

Ward: **Time:**   **Inspections by:**   **Total:**

Project	Location	Content	Points inspections	Scoring criteria	Implement	Not implemented	Problem	Score
Hospital ward infection inspection	Treatment room	Using sterile items, placement	1. Sterile items should be placed correctly	2 points				
		Disposal of Medical Waste	1. Tool box should be used correctly	2 points				
			2. Medical waste in yellow bag and temporary storage to the side door of the clean area	2 points				
		Use sharp, no secondary sorting	1. Use sharp, no secondary sorting	2 points				
	Buffer	Goggles pretreatment sterilized	1. Pretreatment goggles in correct position and concentration (1000 mg / L chlorine disinfectant)	2 points				
			2. Goggles correct transport processes, disinfection record	2 points				
		Buffer cleaning and disinfection	1. Buffer walls, floors, the recording surface disinfection	2 points				

Continuous the table

| Ward: | | Time: | | Inspections by: | | | Total: | |
Project	Location	Content	Points inspections	Scoring criteria	Implement	Not implemented	Problem	Score
Hospital ward infection inspection	Buffer	Items placed reasonable	1. Hand disinfectent display	1 point				
			2. Mirror display	1 point				
			3. Trash place	1 point				
	Ward	Environment clean, no garbage piling up	1. Clean environment, timely medical waste treatment	1 point				
		The scope of work of cleaning staff in line with the requirements ward	1. Cleaning staff to do: separate clean sewage, frequency meet the requirements	2 points				
		Use of the disinfectant cleaning staff	1. Disinfectant storage up to standard (the test paper of concentration)	2 points				
		Clean towels used, a sufficient number of towels, Use	1. Towels placed in a proper partition and meet using standard	2 points				

Continuous the table

Ward:		Time:		Inspections by:			Total:	
Project	Location	Content	Points inspections	Scoring criteria	Implement	Not implemented	Problem	Score
Hospital ward infection inspection	Ward	Cleaning staff whether hoarding ward cartons and other trash	1. Other auxiliary space between Ward and other temporary storage without extraneous items pile up	2 points				
		Equipment and instruments disinfection implementation (staff, frequency, system, concentration)	1. Equipment disinfection recording	2 points				
		Medical waste collection implement (e.g. using sharps containers stamped and sealed when upto 3/4)	1. Double sealed medical waste collection, and has transfer record	2 points				

Continuous the table

Project	Location	Content	Points inspections	Scoring criteria	Implement	Not implemented	Problem	Score
Hospital ward infection inspection	Ward	Implement the transfer record of medical waste	1. Double sealed medical waste collection, and has transfer record	2 points				
		Ward negative pressure meter operates normally	1. Ward negative pressure meter operates normally (5Pa)	1 point				
	Management	Monitoring the completion of the nosocomial infection quality control	1. Wear off indicators monitoring records protective equipment, hand hygiene, etc.	2 points				
		Training	1. Ward nosocomial infection training records, attendance sheets, training assessment	2 points				

Ward:　　Time:　　Inspections by:　　Total:

Continuous the table

Ward:		Time:		Inspections by:				Total:	
Project	Location	Content	Points inspections	Scoring criteria	Implement	Not implemented	Problem	Score	
Hospital ward infection inspection	Management	Contingency plans: whether the department has trained personnel to grasp the situation	1. Ward emergency plan and knowledge	2 points					
		Channel management: Personnel restriction in each channel, on and off in specs	1. Each buffer gate long closed	2 points					
			2. The channel door long closed	2 points					
		UV: the timing, disinfection, registration	1. UV lamp, air disinfection machine record	1 point					

Appendix 5   Cleaning and Disinfection Checklist of Wuhan Leishenshan Hospital

Ward name: Check date: Examiner:

Is there a cleaning and disinfection system?	☐ yes ☐ no
Whether you have received pre–job training?	☐ yes ☐ no
Does the concentration of the cleaning disinfectant meet the requirements?	☐ yes ☐ no
Whether the cleaning tools are differentiated and divided into different colors?	☐ yes ☐ no
Are there sufficient numbers of cleaning towels?	☐ yes ☐ no
Are there sufficient numbers of towels for floor cleaning?	☐ yes ☐ no
Frequency of daily disinfection in isolated wards	☐ 1 time / day ☐ 2 times / day ☐ 3 times and above / day
Scope of cleaning	☐ public area ground ☐ Ward floor ☐ surfaces of public areas such as desktops ☐ surfaces of objects in ward ☐ bed rails, bedside tables, etc. ☐ equipment surfaces
Surface cleaning tools	☐ duster cloth ☐ disposable wipes
Is there a secondary immersion of the cleaning tools?	☐ yes ☐ no
Whether the equipment is routinely cleaned and disinfected?	☐ yes ☐ no
Frequency of equipment disinfection	☐ once / day ☐ twice / day ☐ 3 times and above / day

Continuous the table

Concentration of the disinfectant used for cleaning the equipment	□ Chlorine disinfectant
	  ○ 500mg/L
	  ○ 500 ~ 1000mg/L
	  ○ 1000 ~ 2000mg/L
	  ○ 2000mg / L or more
	□ 75% alcohol
	□ disinfection wipes
	□ others

Appendix 6　Guideline for Individual Protection in Wuhan Leishenshan Hospital (First Edition)

	Area	Working description	Surgical masks	Medical respirators	Caps	Gloves	Goggles/face shields	Scrubs	Shoe covers	Protective gowns	Protective boots	Barrier gowns	White coats	Supplementary
Non-medical behavior areas	Non-medical areas, like office and living area, include office, material warehouse, hotel, health care access/corridor and other clean areas		✓							×	×	×	×	
Contaminated areas outside ward	Direction to contamination outside wards according to sketch map of contaminated area	Staffs responsible for patient transportation, examination out of ward, sending specimens, medical waste transfer, domestic garbage transfer etc.		✓	✓	✓	✓ (When necessary)			✓	✓			Staffs in this area are not allowed to walk back to the clean area, who should wear or take off protective gear in specified area according to the designated rules

Continuous the table

Area	Working description	Surgical masks	Medical respirators	Caps	Gloves	Goggles/face shields	Scrubs	Shoe covers	Protective gowns	Protective boots	Barrier gowns	White coats	Supplementary
Clean areas outside ward	According to sketch map of contaminated area, specifically refer to doctor office, nursing station, therapeutic room, changing room, etc.	√	√ (When necessary)	√			√				√ (When necessary)	√ (When necessary)	Staffs in this area are not allowed to go out directly wearing protective gowns or to the non-medical areas

Continuous the table

Area	Working description	Surgical masks	Medical respirators	Caps	Gloves	Goggles/face shields	Scrubs	Shoe covers	Protective gowns	Protective boots	Barrier gowns	White coats	Supplementary
Potentially/contaminated areas	According to sketch map of contaminated area, specifically refer to wards and corridors, etc.	√ (When necessary)	√	√	√	√ (When necessary)	√	√	√ (When necessary)	√	√	√ (When necessary)	Staffs in this area are not allowed to walk back to the clean areas in protective gowns, but only in conditions of taking off protective gear in strict orders according to the designated rules. When accompanying patient to examination, patient access should be used

Notes: √ recommendated; × forbidden

Appendix 7　Information Verification Mechanism for Nosocomial Infection Outbreak Report at Wuhan Leishenshan Hospital

To improve the capacity of our hospitals to identify and handle outbreaks of nosocomial infection, as well as prevent spread and guarantee occupational safety for medical staff, we have developed an information verification mechanism in this outbreak report.

1. System of Verification

1.1 In case the managing physician and nurse in charge of infectious diseases fing more than three cases infected with the same pathogen within a short time, and the drug resistance spectrum among the cases is highly identical or completely consistent, the managing physician should judge whether the outbreak of nosocomial infection is a hospital infection outbreak or not. If the answer is "yes" or "highly suspected", it should be reported immediately to the director of the department, and the director organized other people to check above cases and re-judged whether it is an outbreak of nosocomial infection. If the cases are still judged to be "yes" or "highly suspected", the nosocomial infection management team was immediately informed by telephone.

1.2 If the sporadic case monitoring team, multidrug-resistant bacteria monitors and community managers of nosocomial infection management team find that more than three cases of infection of the same pathogen occur in a department, they should report to the head of the nosocomial infection management team.

1.3 Once the outbreaks or suspected outbreaks of nosocomial infection is reported through the relevant channels, the nosocomial infection management team should constitute a team of epidemiological investigators to immediately carry out verification work. The nosocomial infection management team should facilitate the inspection staff according to the seriousness of the circumstances and the work to be done.

2. Object of Verification

Patients, family members and medical staff with nosocomial infection.

3. Content of Verification

3.1 Check for nosocomial infection.

3.2 Check whether the nosocomial infection occurred is an outbreak.

3.3 Check the patient's name, bed number, admission date, doctor in charge, whether there is an infection, nosocomial infection, the infection site, the pathogen, and the drug resistance.

3.4 Check the name of the family members, whether there is an infection, nosocomial infection, the infection site, the pathogen, and the drug resistance.

3.5 Check the name of the medical staff, the department, whether there is an infection, nosocomial infection, the infection site, the pathogen, and the drug resistance.

4.Methods of Verification

4.1 System check: Inquire the patient information through the nosocomial infection report of HIS and inquire the drug resistance of the pathogen through LIS.

4.2 Field check: Visit the clinical department to investigate the information about the outbreak of nosocomial infection.

5.Main Responsibilities of Relevant Departments

5.1 Clinical department: Provide network reports of nosocomial infection cases and telephone reports of outbreaks or suspected outbreaks of nosocomial infection.

5.2 Nosocomial infection management team: Organize and complete the investigation of nosocomial infection outbreak under the leadership of nosocomial infection committee, including timely screening of nosocomial infection cases in the nosocomial infection reporting system, determining whether it is a nosocomial infection outbreak or suspected outbreak, completing the homology identification of pathogens, etc. In the event of an outbreak, timely emergency plans should be initiated to control the spread of the outbreak.

5.3 Infectious physician: Responsible for verifying the diagnosis of nosocomial infection.

6.Work Requirements

Each department should attach great importance to this process, the nosocomial infection management team should set up a special person to be responsible for ensuring the authenticity and reliability of relevant information.

Appendix 8　Outbreak Case Survey Form

(Suspected) Case Investigation of Nosocomial Infection

A.1 General Information

A.1.1 Patient name：　　　　　Parent's name (if child, please fill in)

A.1.2 Patient ID:

A.1.3 Gender：☐ male　☐ female

A.1.4 Age：　years（months）

A.2 Discovery / Reporting Information

A.2.1 Case ID：

A.2.2 The infection occurred department：

A.2.3 Departments where the patient is admitted：

A.2.4 Date of onset：year　month　day

A.2.5 Discovery time：year　month　day

A.2.6 Diagnosis and site of infection：

A.3 Onset and Consultation

A.3.1 Admission date：year　month　day

A.3.2 Possible causes of infection：

A.3.3 Primary diseases：

A.4 Clinical Manifestation

A.4.1 Clinical symptoms：

A.4.2 Clinical signs：

A.4.3 Microbiological inspection results and dates：

A.5 High Risk Factors and Exposure

A.5.1 Ward environment：☐ type I　☐ type II　☐ type III

A.5.2 Health care：nurse in charge　　day care nurse　　doctor in charge

Wash hands before or after each contact with the patient or use a quick hand sanitizer ☐ yes ☐ no　Attendance of medical staff:

A.5.3 Whether the surrounding patients have similar clinical symptoms and signs: ☐ yes ☐ no

A.5.4 Patient-related medical devices: Before and after use
□ disinfection □ sterilization

A.5.5 Results of recent environmental spot checks: air: object
surface: staff hands:

A.5.6 Is there a suspicious use of disinfectant: lot number:

A.5.7 Is there a suspicious intravenous injection: lot number:

A.5.8 The number of patients in this group: , Case number of the patient: ,
Possible sources of infection for the patient: □ patient itself   □ other patients
□ medical staff □ medical instruments □ hospital environment □ food □ medicine
Rvisitor □ assistant □ unknown source of infection □ other

A.5.9 Survey of patient susceptibility factors

Name of surgery: Emergency: yes □   no □

Date of surgery: Participants: Surgery duration: hours   minutes

Surgical implant: yes □   no □

Surgical incision type: clean □   clean-contaminated □ contaminated □
infected □

Anesthesia (ASA) score:

Surgery grade: grade I □ grade II □ grade III □ grade IV □ grade V□

Anesthesia: general anesthesia □   epidural anesthesia □ lumbar anesthesia □

Diabetes   □ Immunodeficiency   □ Urinary cannula □ duration (   )
Tumor □ Immunosuppressant □ Arteriovenous cannula □ duration (   )
Coma □ Hypoproteinemia □ Place of the drainage tube (   ) duration (   )
Liver cirrhosis □ WBC < 1.5×10^9/L □ Use of glucocorticoid (   )
Radiotherapy □ Chemotherapy □ Tracheotomy □ yes □ no duration (   ) Using
a ventilator   □ yes   □ no duration (   ) Asthma □ Coronary heart disease □
Chronic kidney disease □   Chronic bronchitis □ Other chronic lung diseases □
Other chronic diseases □

A.6 Patient Lifestyle, Past Health History

A.6.1 Wash hands before meals: □ everytime   □ occasionally   □ never
□ other

A.6.2 Other infection before this infection ☐ yes ☐ no, Site of infection:

A.7 Application of antibacterial drugs

type: name: days used / start and end date

A.8 Laboratory Tests

A.8.1 Infection-related indicators: Blood routine test: ; CRP: ;PCT: ；
other:

A.8.2 Investigation of serological and pathogenic tests

Specimen type   Sampling time   Test items   Test method   Test unit
Results

Note: Specimen types include throat swabs, sputum, blood, urine, stool, secretions, and other clinical specimens related to the infection.

A.9 Outcome and Final Diagnosis

A.9.1 Final diagnosis: ☐ confirmed case   ☐ suspected case   ☐ clinically diagnosed case ☐ excluded case

A.9.2 Diagnostic unit:

A.9.3 Outcome: ☐ fully recovered, discharge date: month   day ☐ death, date of death: month   day cause of death: ☐ other

A.10 Other matters to be recorded

Increase or decrease the content of the case list according to the actual situation. E.g. if it is suspected to be related to anesthetics and disinfectants, the relevant information of the anesthetics and disinfectants should be recorded, as well as the follow-up of the remaining anesthetics and disinfectants for testing. If it is suspected to be related to the implant, information about the implant and testing of the same batch of implants should be recorded. Relevant information should be traced if suspected to be related to Disinfection Supply Center (CSSD).

A.11 Survey Unit, Personnel and Time

A.11.1 Survey unit:

A.11.2 Investigator signature:

A.11.3 Investigation time: month   day—— month   day